MILITARY AND VETERAN ISSUES

VETERAN INJURIES, DISORDERS AND MEDICAL CARE SERVICE

MILITARY AND VETERAN ISSUES

Additional books in this series can be found on Nova's website under the Series tab.

Additional E-books in this series can be found on Nova's website under the E-book tab.

MILITARY AND VETERAN ISSUES

VETERAN INJURIES, DISORDERS AND MEDICAL CARE SERVICE

JESSICA MICHAELS
AND
JESSE E. LEVINE
EDITORS

Nova Science Publishers, Inc.
New York

Library of Congress Cataloging-in-Publication Data

ISBN: 978-1-62081-302-7

Published by Nova Science Publishers, Inc. † New York

CONTENTS

PREFACE

A broad range of medical care services and benefits are offered to veterans of the U.S. Armed Forces. This book examines a variety of medical conditions which afflict veterans, basic eligibility criteria for VA administered veterans' benefits, types of medical care offered and social policy considerations. Topics include suicide and VA prevention efforts; PTSD and substance use among Operation Enduring Freedom (OEF) and Operation Iraqi Freedom (OIF) veterans; traumatic brain injury among veterans; veterans' mental health; VA community living centers; outpatient clinics; and veterans' medical care appropriations.

Chapter 1- A broad range of benefits are offered to veterans of the U.S. Armed Forces and to certain members of their families by the U.S. Department of Veterans Affairs (VA). Among these benefits are various types of financial assistance, including monthly cash payments to disabled veterans, health care, education, and housing benefits. Basic criteria must be met to be eligible to receive any of the benefits administered by the VA.

For a former servicemember to receive certain VA benefits, the person must have active U.S. military service for a minimum period of time and meet nature of discharge requirements. Some members of the National Guard and reserve components have difficulty meeting the active duty and length of service requirements. However, a member of the National Guard or reserve components who is activated for federal military service and serves the full period of activation is considered a veteran for purposes of VA benefits.

The GI Bill Improvement Act of 1977 (P.L. 95-202) recognized the service of one group of civilians, the Women's Air Forces Service Pilots, as active service for benefits administered by the VA, and it also established that the Secretary of Defense could determine that service for the Armed Forces by a group of civilians, or contractors, be considered active service for benefits administered by the VA.

This report examines the basic eligibility criteria for VA administered veterans' benefits, including the issue of eligibility of members of the National Guard and reserve components.

Chapter 2- The United States has provided benefits in varying degrees to those who have worn the uniform and suffered disabilities in service to the nation. In general, a veteran is entitled to compensation for disabilities incurred in or aggravated during active military, naval, or air service. It should be noted that not all persons who served in the military are considered veterans for purposes of veterans benefits. Veterans could meet the burden of proving that their disabilities are service-connected through their military records, which may clearly describe and document the circumstances and medical treatment for an injury or an illness incurred while in service as well as any resulting disability. However, where the manifestation of the disability is remote from the veteran's service and any relationship between the disability and service is not readily apparent, the burden of proving service connection can be a challenge. In such circumstances, Congress and the Department of Veterans Affairs (VA) have relied on presumptions. In the context of VA claims adjudication, a presumption could be seen as a procedure to relieve veterans of the burden to prove that a disability or illness was caused by a specific exposure that occurred during service in the Armed Forces. When a disease is designated as presumptively service-connected, the individual veteran does not need to prove that the disease was incurred during service.

Chapter 3- On May 10, 2011, the Ninth Circuit Court of Appeals ruled against the Department of Veterans Affairs (VA) in a case brought by two nonprofit veterans advocacy groups, Veterans for Common Sense and Veterans United for Truth. The ruling criticized the VA's mental health services, among other things. This has intensified interest in veterans' mental health, already a topic of ongoing concern to Members of Congress and their constituents.

This brief report addresses three relevant topics: suicide, posttraumatic stress disorder (PTSD), and substance use disorders. Using data from the VA, it answers two questions about each topic: (1) How many veterans of Operations Enduring Freedom and Iraqi Freedom (OEF/OIF) are affected? and (2) What is the VA doing, in terms of screening, prevention, and treatment?

Chapter 4- Traumatic Brain Injury (TBI) has been defined as "an alteration in brain function, or other evidence of brain pathology, caused by an external force." In the general population, TBI results mainly from falls, motor vehicle/traffic accidents, assaults, and other instances in which the head is struck by or strikes against an object. In military servicemembers, TBI may also result from improvised explosive devices, mortars, grenades, bullets, or mines.

Traumatic brain injury has become known as a "signature wound" of Operation Enduring Freedom (OEF) and Operation Iraqi Freedom (OIF), because the incidence of TBI is higher in these conflicts than it has been in previous conflicts. As of FY2010, 1.25 million OEF/OIF veterans have left active duty and became eligible for Department of Veterans Affairs (VA) health care; half of them have obtained VA health care; and 45,606 have been diagnosed with TBI-related conditions at VA medical facilities. The total number of OEF/OIF veterans with TBI is not known, in part because some OEF/OIF veterans have not accessed VA health care services.

Chapter 5- Responsibility for prevention of veteran suicide lies primarily with the Veterans Health Administration (VHA), within the Department of Veterans Affairs (VA). The VHA Strategic Plan for Suicide Prevention is based on a public health framework, which has three major components: (1) surveillance, (2) risk and protective factors, and (3) prevention interventions.

No nationwide surveillance system exists for suicide among all veterans; therefore, the actual incidence of suicide among veterans is not known. Surveillance, or systematic collection of data on completed (i.e., fatal) suicides, is essential to define the scope of the problem (i.e., the suicide rate among veterans), identify characteristics associated with higher or lower risk of suicide, and track changes in the suicide rate over time to evaluate suicide prevention interventions. In the absence of a nationwide surveillance system for veteran suicide, the VHA is attempting to determine the rate of suicide among veterans in two ways, both in collaboration with the Centers for Disease Control and Prevention (CDC).

Information collected in surveillance is used to identify suicide risk factors (i.e., characteristics associated with higher rates of suicide) and protective factors (i.e., characteristics associated with lower rates of suicide). This is essential in order to design interventions that reduce risk factors and/or increase protective factors, thus lowering overall risk of suicide. Risk factors are also helpful in identifying at-risk groups or individuals so that interventions can be delivered to the people who need them most. Within the VHA, this research is supported by the Office of Research and Development; a Center of Excellence in suicide prevention; and a Mental Illness Research, Education, and Clinical Center on suicide prevention.

Chapter 6- In fiscal year 2010, the Department of Veterans Affairs (VA) provided health care to about 5.2 million veterans. Recent legislation has increased many Operations Enduring Freedom (OEF) and Iraqi Freedom (OIF) veterans' priority for accessing VA's health care, and concerns have been raised about the extent to which VA is providing mental health care to eligible veterans of all eras. There also are concerns that barriers may hinder some veterans from accessing needed mental health care.

GAO was asked to provide information on veterans who receive mental health care from VA. In this report, GAO provides information on (1) how many veterans received mental health care from VA from fiscal years 2006 through 2010, (2) key barriers that may hinder veterans from accessing mental health care from VA, and (3) VA efforts to increase veterans' access to VA mental health care. GAO obtained data from VA's Northeast Program Evaluation Center (NEPEC) on the number of veterans who received mental health care from VA. The number of veterans represents a unique count of veterans; veterans were counted only once, even if they received care multiple times during a fiscal year or across the 5-year period. GAO also reviewed literature published from 2006 to 2011, reviewed VA documents, and interviewed officials from VA and veterans service organizations (VSO).

Chapter 7- The Department of Veterans Affairs (VA) annually provides care to more than 46,000 elderly and disabled veterans in 132 VA-operated nursing homes, called community living centers (CLC). After media reports of problems with the care delivered to veterans in CLCs, VA contracted with the Long Term Care Institute, Inc. (LTCI), a nonprofit organization that surveys nursing homes, to conduct in-depth reviews of CLCs in 2007-2008 and again in 2010-2011. GAO was asked to evaluate VA's approach to managing veterans' quality of care and quality of life in CLCs. This report examines (1) VA's response to and resolution of LTCI-identified deficiencies and (2) information VA collects about the quality of care and quality of life in CLCs and how VA uses it to identify and manage risks. To do this work, GAO interviewed officials from VA headquarters, examined all 116 2007-2008 and 67 2010-2011 LTCI reviews, and analyzed 50 CLCs' corrective action plans for 2007-2008 and 23 such plans for 2010-2011.

Chapter 8- In the early 1990s, the Veterans Health Administration (VHA)—one of the three administrations of the Department of Veterans Affairs (VA)—began developing a strategy to expand its capacity to provide outpatient primary care, especially for veterans who had to travel long distances to receive care at VA facilities. To facilitate access to primary care closer to where veterans reside, VHA began implementing a system for approving and establishing Community-Based Outpatient Clinics (CBOCs).

A CBOC is a fixed health care site that is geographically distinct or separate from its parent VA medical facility. A CBOC can be either VA-owned and VA-staffed or contracted to Healthcare Management Organizations (HMO). Regardless of how it is administered, a

CBOC must have the necessary professional medical staff, access to diagnostic testing and treatment capability, and the referral arrangements needed to ensure continuity of health care for current or eligible veteran patients. VA policies require all CBOCs to be operated in a manner that provides veterans with consistent, safe, high-quality health care.

CBOCs are managed at the Veterans Integrated Service Network (VISN) level, and planning and development of a new CBOC is based on the VA's need, available resources, local market circumstances, and veteran preference.

Chapter 9- The Department of Veterans Affairs (VA) provides benefits to veterans who meet certain eligibility criteria. Benefits to veterans range from disability compensation and pensions to hospital and medical care. The VA provides these benefits through three major operating units: the Veterans Health Administration (VHA), the Veterans Benefits Administration (VBA), and the National Cemetery Administration (NCA).

This report focuses on the VHA. The VHA is primarily a direct service provider of primary care, specialized care, and related medical and social support services to veterans through the nation's largest integrated health care system. Veterans generally must enroll in the VA health care system to receive medical care. Eligibility for enrollment is based primarily on previous military service, disability, and income. VA provides free inpatient and outpatient medical care to veterans for service-connected conditions and to low-income veterans for nonservice-connected conditions. The President submitted his FY2012 budget request to Congress on February 14, 2011.

The Administration's FY2012 budget request for VHA (medical services, medical support and compliance, medical facilities, and medical and prosthetic research) was $51.4 billion. The President's budget proposed to set up a $953 million contingency fund that would have provided additional funds up to $953 million to become available for obligation if the Administration determined that additional funds were required due to changes in economic conditions in 2012.

In: Veteran Injuries, Disorders and Medical Care Service ISBN: 978-1-62081-302-7
Editors: Jessica Michaels and Jesse E. Levine

Chapter 1

"Who Is a Veteran?" — Basic Eligibility for Veterans' Benefits*

Christine Scott

Summary

A broad range of benefits are offered to veterans of the U.S. Armed Forces and to certain members of their families by the U.S. Department of Veterans Affairs (VA). Among these benefits are various types of financial assistance, including monthly cash payments to disabled veterans, health care, education, and housing benefits. Basic criteria must be met to be eligible to receive any of the benefits administered by the VA.

For a former servicemember to receive certain VA benefits, the person must have active U.S. military service for a minimum period of time and meet nature of discharge requirements. Some members of the National Guard and reserve components have difficulty meeting the active duty and length of service requirements. However, a member of the National Guard or reserve components who is activated for federal military service and serves the full period of activation is considered a veteran for purposes of VA benefits.

The GI Bill Improvement Act of 1977 (P.L. 95-202) recognized the service of one group of civilians, the Women's Air Forces Service Pilots, as active service for benefits administered by the VA, and it also established that the Secretary of Defense could determine that service for the Armed Forces by a group of civilians, or contractors, be considered active service for benefits administered by the VA.

This report examines the basic eligibility criteria for VA administered veterans' benefits, including the issue of eligibility of members of the National Guard and reserve components.

---

* This is an edited, reformatted and augmented version of the Congressional Research Service Publication, CRS Report for Congress R42324, dated January 23, 2012.

Introduction

A broad range of benefits are offered to veterans of the U.S. Armed Forces and to certain members of their families by the U.S. Department of Veterans Affairs (VA). Among these benefits are various types of financial assistance, including monthly cash payments to disabled veterans, health care, education, and housing benefits. Basic criteria must be met to be eligible to receive any of the benefits administered by the VA.

This report focuses upon the basic eligibility/entitlement requirements for former servicemembers for veterans' benefits administered by the VA. Certain VA benefits are available to current servicemembers, and the eligibility requirements for those benefits are not a component of this report.

The VA uses a two-step process to evaluate claims for benefits. First, the claimant must demonstrate that he or she is *eligible*. That is, the claimant must prove that he or she is a bona fide veteran and verify certain related matters. In this sense, the eligibility relates to the veteran's general qualification(s) for the benefit(s). Second, the veteran must prove *entitlement* to the particular benefit being sought.[1]

Who Is a Veteran?

To be eligible for most VA benefits, the claimant must be a veteran or, in some circumstances, the survivor or the dependent of a veteran. By statute, a "veteran" is defined as a "person who served in the active military, naval, or air service, and who was discharged or released therefrom under conditions other than dishonorable."[2]

In evaluating the evidence to determine whether the applicant is a "veteran" for the purposes of VA benefits, the VA relies upon military department service records. The VA is bound by information that the service documents contain.[3] Generally speaking, the VA findings will be in accord with the information contained in the applicant's military service records.[4]

Such records may include an original military service record; a copy issued by the military service with the certification that it is a true document; or a copy submitted by an accredited agent, attorney, or service representative with special training, who certifies that it is a copy of an original military service document or a copy of a copy of such a document.[5] In addition to meeting these criteria, the document must contain data regarding the length, time, and character of the service, and the VA must believe that the document is genuine and accurate.[6] If the claimant does not provide the requisite documentation or other evidence, or the submitted documentation does not meet the requirements, the VA must seek to verify the applicant's military service directly from the appropriate military service.[7]

Active Service

An applicant must have "active military, naval, or air service" to be considered a veteran for most VA benefits.[8] However, not all types of service are considered active military service for this purpose.[9]

In general, active service means full-time service, other than active duty for training, as a member of the Army, Navy, Air Force, Marine Corps, Coast Guard, or as a commissioned officer of the Public Health Service, the Environmental Science Services Administration or the National Oceanic and Atmospheric Administration, or its predecessor, the Coast and Geodectic Survey.

Active service also includes a period of active duty for training during which the person was disabled or died from an injury or disease incurred or aggravated in the line of duty[10] and any period of inactive duty for training during which the person was disabled or died from an injury incurred or aggravated in the line of duty or from certain health conditions incurred during the training.[11]

Additional circumstances of service, and whether they are deemed to be active military service, are set out in law.[12] For example, if on authorized travel to and from the performance of active duty training or inactive duty for training, a person is disabled or dies while proceeding directly to or returning from such duty, the duty will be considered to be active duty for training or inactive duty for training.[13]

The determination of whether a claimant has met the "active service" requirement may not be a simple process. It is possible that the claimant and the VA may have to scrutinize the claimant's service record(s) to determine whether the claimant's service fits into one of the many categories of active service, or whether an exception has been made for his or her service, so that it is considered to be active service for the purposes of veterans' benefits. In addition, a claimant may have more than one period of service, which may further complicate the determination.

Length of Service

Prior to September 8, 1980, there was no minimum length of service necessary to be considered a veteran for most VA benefits. However, for an individual who enlisted after September 8, 1980, there are now certain minimum length of service requirements. The general requirement is either 24 months of continuous active duty or the "full period" for which the servicemember was called or ordered to active duty.[14]

Several exceptions exist to this general rule. For example, service-connected disability compensation benefits are exempt from the minimum active duty requirements. Thus, a veteran with a disease or injury incurred during active service should almost always be able to receive service-connected compensation for his or her condition or disability.[15] Other exceptions to the minimum service requirements include claims for VA life insurance benefits,[16] hardship discharges,[17] and persons retired or separated from service because of a service-related disability.[18]

If the former servicemember does not fall within the 24 months of active duty or the "full period" of active duty, or within one of the statutory exceptions, then the veteran has not completed a minimum period of active duty and is "not eligible for any benefit under Title 38,

United States Code or under any law administered by the Department of Veterans Affairs based on that period of active service."[19]

Discharge Criteria

The statutory definition of "veteran" requires that the individual be discharged or released from military service "under conditions other than dishonorable."[20] There are currently five types of discharges issued by the military services: (1) honorable discharge (HD), (2) discharge under honorable conditions (UHC) or general discharge (GD), (3) discharge under other than honorable conditions (UOTHC) or undesirable discharge (UD), (4) bad conduct discharge (BCD), and (5) dishonorable discharge (DD).[21]

The language of the statute does not precisely match the current categories of the discharges, and the VA often determines on a case-by-case basis whether the claimant's discharge satisfies any of the criteria and which category of discharge applies. In most cases, the VA considers honorable discharges and discharges under honorable conditions to fall within the "conditions other than dishonorable" category, and will usually qualify the claimant as a veteran under the first step of the eligibility test.[22] Usually, honorable and general discharges qualify a veteran for most benefits.[23]

A bad conduct discharge from a special court-martial and other discharges made under other than honorable conditions may or may not disqualify the claimant from being considered a veteran for purposes of benefits eligibility.[24] In the case of such a discharge, the VA will make a special "character of service determination," based on the particular facts in the claimant's case. On this basis, the VA will determine whether the veteran was separated from service under "dishonorable conditions" or under "other than dishonorable conditions." The VA will review the entire period of the claimant's enlistment(s) to assess the quality of the service and to determine whether it is sufficient to deserve the award of veterans' benefits.[25] If a claimant has served more than one period of enlistment, he or she may have two or more different discharge categories.

Dishonorable and bad conduct discharges issued by general courts-martial may bar VA benefits. Veterans in prison and parolees may be eligible for certain VA benefits and must contact the VA to determine eligibility. VA benefits will not be provided to any veteran or dependent wanted for an outstanding felony warrant.

Certain exceptions permit the award of VA benefits, even if the character of the discharge would ordinarily bar VA benefits. For example, if it is determined that the claimant was insane at the time of the offense leading up to the discharge, the claimant may be granted VA benefits. There does not need to be a direct connection between the insanity and the misconduct.[26]

Whether the Military Service Was during a Time of War[27]

All military service is classified as either wartime or peacetime service. Whether a veteran has served during a time of war may impact his or her potential VA benefits. For example, the Improved Pension benefit for low- income veterans who are either elderly or non-service-connected disabled veterans, is only for veterans with wartime service.[28]

Congress has set out the periods of "wartime" for the purposes of veterans' benefits.[29] To be considered to have "served during wartime" by the VA, a veteran does not have to have served in an actual combat zone, but during the specified periods of war set out below. Those time periods not designated by Congress as "wartime" are considered to be "peacetime." If a veteran served his or her duty partly during wartime and partly during peacetime, the veteran would meet the "wartime" criteria if he or she served 90 consecutive days, at least one day of which occurred during a period designated as wartime.

Following is a list of those periods of "wartime" designated by Congress:

- *Indian Wars*—January 1, 1817, through December 31, 1898[30]
- *Spanish-American War*—April 21, 1898, through July 4, 1902[31]
- *Mexican Border Period*—May 19, 1916, though April 5, 1917[32]
- *World War I*—April 6, 1917, through November 11, 1918; extended to April 1, 1920; by regulation extended to July 1, 1921, under certain specific conditions[33]
- *World War II*—December 7, 1941, through December 31, 1946; extended to July 25, 1947[34]
- *Korean Conflict*—June 27, 1950, through January 31, 1955[35]
- *Vietnam Era*—August 5, 1964, through May 7, 1975[36]
- *Persian Gulf War*—August 2, 1990, through a date to be prescribed by Presidential proclamation or law[37]

NATIONAL GUARD AND RESERVE

Two particular elements of the criteria to be a veteran—"active duty" and "length of service"— are often difficult for members of the National Guard and the reserve components to meet. As a result, these servicemembers, having not met the statutory threshold criteria for "veteran," are often not eligible for VA benefits.

In many cases, members of the Guard and the reserves may not have fulfilled the "active duty" requirement. Members of the Guard and reserves who have never been activated for federal active duty military service, and consequently have not served on regular federal active duty, do not meet the active duty requirement for the definition of a veteran for VA benefits.

For other National Guard and reserve members, the two requirements may be met at the same time. An example of this situation would be a Guard or reserve member who was activated for federal military service and served in the Persian Gulf for 12 months. At the end of the activation period, the servicemember would be considered to have served on active duty for that period of time. Serving for the full period of activation also meets the minimum length of service requirement to be a veteran. Otherwise, Guard and reserve duty may not be considered "active duty" for benefits unless the servicemember performing this duty was disabled or died from a disease or injury incurred or aggravated in the line of duty.[38]

Although many National Guard and reserve members may not appear to be eligible "veterans" for the purposes of VA benefits, certain exceptions and special circumstances may exist, which add to the complexity of the eligibility determination. For example, under certain conditions Guard and reserve members may be eligible for education benefits (through the

Reserve Educational Program or the Post-9/11 GI Bill) and home loans from the VA (with six years of service in the Selected Reserves or National Guard). As each servicemember's military service may be different, and therefore may fit within certain case categories or exceptions, eligibility is usually determined by the VA on a case-by-case basis after reviewing the individual servicemember's military service records.

CIVILIAN GROUPS

The GI Bill Improvement Act of 1977 (P.L. 95-202) recognized the service of one group of civilians, the Women's Air Forces Service Pilots, as active service for benefits administered by the U.S. Department of Veterans Affairs. In addition, P.L. 95-202 provided that the Secretary of Defense could determine that service for the Armed Forces by a group of civilians, or contractors, be considered active service for benefits administered by the VA.

Based on the provisions of P.L. 95-202,[39] the Secretary of Defense established that the Secretary of the Air Force would develop and maintain the process to determine if the wartime employment of certain groups of individuals is considered "active duty" military service for the purpose of receiving certain veterans benefits. If these groups of individuals are considered to be "active duty" by the Secretary, they are eligible to receive certain benefits, including health care.[40]

Regulations implementing P.L. 95-202 specify which groups the Secretary has determined were employed in "active duty" service.[41] The regulations also established the Department of Defense Civilian/Military Service Review Board and Advisory Panel to review each application for "active duty" status.[42] Following its review, the board issues a written recommendation to the Secretary as to whether the applicant group should be considered "active duty" for the purposes of the act. The Secretary makes the final decision, based upon the recommendation of the board. Pursuant to this procedure, various groups of persons have been accorded "active duty" status. Among the successful applicants were Women's Air Forces Service Pilots (WASPs), Signal Corps Female Telephone Operators Unit (World War I), Engineer Field Clerks (World War I), Male Civilian Ferry Pilots (World War II), and other groups of employees with war-related occupations.[43] At this time, all of the successful applicants have been civilian groups associated with World War I and World War II.

The regulations concerning the designation of "active duty" status have undergone revision over the years. Changes and clarification to the regulations implemented in 1989 "stem from a Federal Court determination [*Schumacher v. Aldridge*][44] that the Department of Defense had failed to clarify factors and criteria in their implementing directive concerning P.L. 95-202."[45] The 1989 regulations remain in effect.

End Notes

[1] For example, to be entitled to receive disability compensation, a veteran must provide sufficient evidence of certain elements (e.g., current diagnosis, medical evidence of an in-service occurrence, and link between the in-service occurrence and the current disability).

[2] 38 U.S.C. § 101(2); 38 C.F.R. § 3.1(d).

[3] Venturella v. Gober, 10 Vet. App. 340, 341-342 (1977); Duro v. Derwinski, 2 Vet. App. 530, 532 (1992).

[4] 38 C.F.R. § 3.203.

[5] 38 C.F.R. § 3.203(a)(1). See CRS Report RS21282, *Military Service Records and Unit Histories: A Guide to Locating Sources*, by Julissa Gomez-Granger and Anne Leland.

[6] 38 C.F.R. § 3.203(a)(2), (3).

[7] Duro, 2 Vet. App. at 532.

[8] 38 U.S.C. § 101(2); 38 C.F.R. § 3.12(a).

[9] For example, National Guard and Reserve duty may not be considered active service unless an individual performing this duty was disabled or died from a disease or injury incurred or aggravated in the line of duty. (38 U.S.C. § 101(24); 38 C.F.R. § 3.6(a)).

[10] Active duty for training is a tour of active duty that is used for training members of reserve and other components to fill the Armed Forces during time of war or national emergency. Active duty for training has been determined to mean (1) full-time duty for training performed by Reservists (38 U.S.C. § 101(22)(A); 38 C.F.R. § 3.6(c)(1)); (2) full-time duty for training purposes as a commissioned officer in the Reserved Corps of the Public Health Service (38 U.S.C. § 101(22)(B); 38 C.F.R. § 3.6(c)(2)); (3) full-time training duty by members of the Air or Army National Guard of any state (38 U.S.C. § 101(22)(C); 38 C.F.R. § 3.6(c)(3)); (4) duty by members of the Senior ROTC program on field training or a practice cruise (38 U.S.C. § 101 (22)(D); 38 C.F.R. § 3.6(c)(4)); and (5) authorized travel to and from duty for training (38 U.S.C. § 101(22)(E); 38 C.F.R. § 3.6(c)(6)).

[11] 38 U.S.C. § 101(24). Inactive duty for training has been defined to mean (1) duty, other than full-time duty, for Reservists (38 U.S.C. § 101(23)(A); 38 C.F.R. § 3.6(d)(1)); (2) other duties authorized for Reservists performed on a voluntary basis (38 U.S.C. § 101(23)(B); 38 C.F.R. § 3.6(d)(2)); (3) training (other than active duty for training) by a member of, or applicant for membership in, Senior ROTC (38 U.S.C. § 101(23)(C); 38 C.F.R. § 3.6(d)(3)); and (4) for the members of the Air or Army National Guard of any state, such training means duty other than full-time duty (38 U.S.C. § 101(23); 38 C.F.R. § 3.6(d)(4)).

[12] 38 U.S.C. §§ 101, 106.

[13] 38 U.S.C. § 106(d); 38 C.F.R. § 3.6(e).

[14] 38 U.S.C. § 5303A(b); 38 C.F.R. § 3.12a(a)(1).

[15] 38 U.S.C. § 5303A(b)(3)(C); 38 C.F.R. § 3.12a(d)(4).

[16] 38 U.S.C. § 5303A(b)(3)(E); 38 C.F.R. § 3.12a(d)(5).

[17] 38 U.S.C. § 5303A(b)(3)(A); 38 C.F.R. § 3.12a(d)(1).

[18] 38 U.S.C. § 5303A(b)(3)(B); 38 C.F.R. § 3.12a(d)(2).

[19] 38 U.S.C. § 5303A(b)(1); 38 C.F.R. § 3.12a(b).

[20] 38 U.S.C. § 101(2); 38 C.F.R. § 3.12(a).

[21] Barton F. Stichman et al., *Veterans Benefits Manual*, at § 2.2.1 (Cited to afterward as "Veterans Benefits Manual").

[22] Ibid.

[23] Ibid.

[24] Ibid.

[25] Ibid.

[26] 38 U.S.C. § 5303(b).

[27] See CRS Report RS21405, *U.S. Periods of War and Dates of Current Conflicts*, by Barbara Salazar Torreon.

[28] 38 U.S.C. § 1521(j).

[29] 38 U.S.C. § 101 (6)-(11); 38 C.F.R. § 3.2.

[30] See 38 C.F.R. § 3.2(a).

[31] 38 U.S.C. § 101(6); 38 C.F.R. § 3.2(b).

[32] 38 U.S.C. § 101(30); 38 C.F.R. § 3.2(h).

[33] 38 U.S.C. § 101(7); 38 C.F.R. § 3.2(c).

[34] 38 U.S.C. § 101(8); 38 C.F.R. § 3.2(d).

[35] 38 U.S.C. § 101(9); 38 C.F.R. § 3.2(e).

[36] 38 U.S.C. § 101(29); 38 C.F.R. § 3.2(f). Military personnel who served in the Republic of Vietnam between February 28, 1961, and May 7, 1975, are also considered to have served during the Vietnam Era.

[37] 38 U.S.C. §§ 101(33), 1501(4); 38 C.F.R. §§ 3.2(I), 3.3(a)(3), 3.17, 3.54(a)(3)(viii). At the present time, no termination date has been established.

[38] 38 U.S.C. § 101(21)(A); 38 C.F.R. § 3.6(a). Inactive duty would include duty other than full-time duty, such as weekend assignments or part-time details.

[39] 38 U.S.C. § 106 note.

[40] See 38 C.F.R. § 3.7.

[41] 32 C.F.R. § 47. See 38 C.F.R. § 3.7 for those groups that have been so designated.

[42] The applications are usually submitted by representatives of the employment group.

[43] 38 C.F.R. § 3.7.

[44] 665 F.Supp. 41 (D.D.C. 1987).

[45] 54 *Fed.* Reg. 39,991 (September 29, 1989).

In: Veteran Injuries, Disorders and Medical Care Service ISBN: 978-1-62081-302-7
Editors: Jessica Michaels and Jesse E. Levine

Chapter 2

VETERANS AFFAIRS: PRESUMPTIVE SERVICE CONNECTION AND DISABILITY COMPENSATION[*]

Sidath Viranga Panangala, Christine Scott, Douglas Reid Weimer and Umar Moulta-Ali

SUMMARY

The legislative history of veterans' disease presumptions dates back to 1921 when Congress established a presumption of service connection with an amendment (P.L. 67-47) to the War Risk Insurance Act (P.L. 63-193). It established presumptions of service connection for tuberculosis and neuropsychiatric disease (known today as psychosis) occurring within two years of separation from active duty military service. In the following years, additions to the presumptive list were made by regulation, executive order, and legislation. In the past 22 years, Congress has on three separate occasions created presumptive programs for three distinct groups of veterans: the so-called atomic veterans, who were exposed to radiation from above-ground nuclear tests and the atomic bombs detonated in Japan; Vietnam veterans; and Gulf War veterans. In addition, Congress has added certain disease conditions to the list of presumptions for specific groups of veterans such as former prisoners of war (POWs).

In 1991, the Agent Orange Act (P.L. 102-4) established for Vietnam veterans a presumption of a service connection for diseases associated with exposure to Agent Orange and other herbicides. For the first time, this act required the VA to contract with the Institute of Medicine (IOM) to conduct, every two years, a scientific review of the evidence linking certain medical conditions to herbicide exposure. The VA was instructed to use the IOM's findings, and other evidence, to issue regulations establishing a presumption for any disease for which there is scientific evidence of an association with herbicide exposure.

However, since an increasing proportion of service-connected disability compensation is paid through a presumptive decision-making process, some have raised several policy questions with regard to the current process. This report discusses presumptive service

---

[*] This is an edited, reformatted and augmented version of the Congressional Research Service Publication, CRS Report for Congress R41405, dated March 28, 2011.

connection, its legislative history, and current challenges in making evidence-based determinations of presumptions. It also discusses the Agent Orange Act (P.L. 102-4) and suggests implications of the process established by the act for future presumptive service-connected determinations.

INTRODUCTION

Beginning with the early colonial settlements of America, the nation has provided benefits in varying degrees to those who have worn the uniform and suffered physical disabilities in service to the nation—sacrifices that are inherent to the profession of arms. In 1718, for instance, the colony of Rhode Island enacted legislation that provided benefits not only to every officer, soldier, or sailor who served in the colony's armed services, but also to the wives, children, parents, and other relations who had been dependent upon a slain servicemember. "The physically disabled were to have their wounds carefully tended and healed at the colony's expense, while at the same time an annual pension was provided to him out of the general treasury sufficient for the maintenance of himself and family, or other dependent relatives."[1] These benefits were continued by the Continental Congress, which passed a resolution on August 26, 1776, providing for disabled veterans to receive half of their monthly pay for life or for as long as their disability existed.[2] From the Revolutionary War to the Global War on Terrorism (GWOT),[3] as the nature of the nation's wars has evolved, and as the needs of each generation of veterans who fought those wars have changed, Congress has debated, legislated, and revised benefits provided to veterans.

In general, veterans are eligible for disability compensation if it can be demonstrated that the disabling condition or illness is linked to military service. Veterans could meet the burden of proving that their disabilities were service-connected through their military records, which may clearly describe and document the circumstances and medical treatment for an injury or an illness incurred while in service as well as any resulting disability.[4] However, where the manifestation of the disabling disease or condition is remote from the veteran's service and any relation between the disability and service is not readily apparent, the burden of proving service connection can be a challenge. In such circumstances, Congress and the Department of Veterans Affairs (VA) have relied on presumptions to ease the burden placed on the veteran. Since the early 1920s, almost every Congress has examined the issue of whether one may presume that a veteran's disability is service-connected when there is no clear evidence to establish an illness or disability is caused or aggravated by a veteran's military service. More recently, Congress and the VA have relied on scientific evidence to establish presumptions. However, when the scientific evidence is incomplete and there is uncertainty on the question of causation or if other factors such as natural aging could also contribute to disease causation, Congress and the VA are faced with the challenge of instituting a transparent and equitable process to establish presumptions to compensate veterans for service-connected conditions.

In the early 1990's at the request of the then Chairman of the Senate Committee on Veterans' Affairs, the VA prepared an analysis tracing the historical development of presumptions of service connection.[5] More recently, at the request of the Veterans' Disability Benefits Commission,[6] the Institute of Medicine (IOM) of the National Academy of Sciences

(NAS) did a comprehensive study evaluating the presumptive disability decision-making process, which was released in 2008.[7] Much of the interest with presumptions has focused on Vietnam veterans' exposure to Agent Orange and its contaminant dioxin.[8] The Veterans' Disability Benefits Commission, in its task assignment to IOM, raised some potential issues with the current process of making presumptions:

> Certain studies (not even necessarily involving veterans), for example, showing that those exposed to [Agent Orange] dioxin have slightly higher rates of diabetes or prostate cancer, have resulted in an inexorable push to compensate all veterans with diabetes/prostate cancer even if it is likely that [Agent Orange] dioxin exposure is a determinative factor in only a small percentage of cases. Since it is impossible to know what role dioxin played in any particular case, all Vietnam veterans with diabetes and prostate cancer have been and are being granted presumptive service connection. Is this presumption fully supported by medical evidence? What amount of increase in occurrence rate is enough to warrant compensation? What approaches could be considered to alleviate this costly result?[9]

Organization of This Report

The purpose of this report is to examine the very complex and sometimes controversial policy issue of establishing presumptive service connection. The material in it is based in large part on VA's "Analysis of Presumptions of Service Connection," and IOM's "Improving the Presumptive Disability Decision-Making Process for Veterans" reports.

In order to provide some context to the discussion of presumptions, the first part of this report briefly discusses disability compensation and the establishment of service connection for veterans claiming disability compensation. The second part provides an overview of the legislative history of establishing presumptive service connection. Since most of the controversy about establishing presumptions of service connection is related to exposure to Agent Orange, the third part of this report examines the establishment of presumptions for conditions related to Agent Orange. This part also provides a historical overview leading up to the passage of the Agent Orange Act of 1991 (P.L. 102-4). The fourth part of the report discusses the passage of the Agent Orange Act, which set forth the current process for establishing presumptions. Lastly, it briefly discusses some options that may assist policy makers in their deliberations to make the presumptive decision-making process more transparent and equitable.

DISABILITY COMPENSATION FOR VETERANS

The purpose of disability compensation is to assist currently disabled veterans whose injuries are connected to military service[10] Although a veteran may have been ill or sustained an injury while in service, the mere fact that this occurred is not compensable.[11] It should also be noted that not all persons who served in the military are considered veterans for purposes of veterans benefits.

Currently, there are five ways to establish that a disability is service-connected:[12]

1. Through direct service connection—that is, the facts, shown by evidence, establish that a particular injury or disease resulting in a disability was incurred while in service in the Armed Forces;[13]
2. Through aggravation during service—that is, a preexisting injury or disease willbe considered to have been aggravated while in service in the Armed Forces;[14]
3. Through proximity—that is, a disability, which is proximately due to, or theresult of a service-connected disease or injury which is itself considered to beservice-connected.[15] An example would be a veteran developing cardiovasculardisease due to a service-connected amputation of a lower limb.
4. Through a finding that the disability was caused by medical care or vocationalrehabilitation provided by the Department of Veterans Affairs (VA)—disabilities caused by VA provided medical care or vocational rehabilitation are treated as ifthey are service-connected.[16]
5. Through the application of statutory presumptions—that is, certain diseases asestablished by law or regulation are considered to have been incurred in or aggravated by service in the Armed Forces even though there is no evidence of such disease during the period of service.[17]

VA has the authority to provide disability compensation to veterans by bypassing the first four criteria.[18] The next section discusses what a presumption is, and provides a brief legislative history of establishing presumptive service connection.

PRESUMPTIVE SERVICE CONNECTION

What Is a Presumption?

In the context of VA claims adjudication, a presumption relieves veterans of the burden to prove that a disability or illness was caused by a specific exposure that occurred during service in the Armed Forces. When a disease is designated as presumptively service-connected, the individual veteran does not need to prove that the disease was incurred during service. In other words, a presumption shifts the burden of proof concerning whether a disease or disability was caused or aggravated due to service from the veteran to the VA. The VA would have to demonstrate that some other intervening event caused the disability in order to rebut the presumption.

Often presumptions are applied to chronic diseases or illnesses that manifest after a period of time (sometimes many years) following service, and that may also occur in individuals who have never served. According to the VA's *Analysis of Presumptions of Service Connection:*

> Generally, a legal presumption is a procedural device that shifts the burden of proof by attaching certain consequences to the establishment of certain basic evidentiary facts. When the party invoking a presumption establishes the basic fact(s) giving rise to the presumption, the burden of proof shifts to the other party to prove nonexistence of the presumed fact. A presumption, as used in the law of evidence, is a direction that if fact A (e.g., manifestation within the specified period of a disease

for which a presumption of service connection is available) is established, then fact B (service connection) may be taken as established, even where there is no specific evidence proving fact B (i.e., no medical evidence of a connection between the veteran's disease and the veteran's military service).[19]

Legislative History of Presumptions

The legislative history of veterans' disease presumptions dates back to 1921 when Congress, to ease the decision-making process in VA disability compensation adjudications, used its authority to establish service connection on a presumptive basis. Below is a synopsis of major legislation.

1920s-1940s

The first legislation that specifically established a presumption of service connection was the amendment of August 9, 1921, (P.L. 67-47) to the War Risk Insurance Act (P.L. 63-193). This amendment, among other things, established presumptions of service connection for active pulmonary tuberculosis and neuropsychiatric disease (later known as psychosis) occurring within two years of separation from active duty military service. Prior to the passage of P.L. 67-47, disability compensation for World War I veterans was payable only for a disability directly related to military service. Broadly, the intent of this liberalization legislation was that "as the period beginning with the end of the war lengthened it became increasingly difficult to establish service connection for some ailments, particularly tuberculosis and neuropsychiatric disease."[20] The amendments to the War Risk Insurance Act also gave the then Veterans Bureau authority to establish rules and regulations to carry out provisions in the act. This allowed the agency to promulgate regulations establishing presumption of service connection for certain diseases. As stated in VA's *Analysis of Presumptions of Service Connection:*

> Regulation No. 11 provided that chronic constitutional diseases, other than active pulmonary tuberculosis or neuropsychiatric disease, becoming manifest within one year following the date of separation from active service would be considered as incurred in service or aggravated by service unless there were affirmative evidence to the contrary or evidence establishing that some intercurrent disease or injury which is a recognized cause of the disorder was suffered between the date of separation from service and the onset of the chronic disease. [21]

The next major piece of legislation that established presumptions of service connection was the World War Veterans Act of 1924 (P.L. 68-242) enacted on June 7, 1924. This act made important changes to existing laws on presumptions related to tuberculosis and mental illness. Among other things, this act added the following three diseases to the list of presumptive diseases: dysentery (amebic) (tropical disease added as chronic disease); paralysis agitans (now known as Parkinson's disease); and encephalitis lethargica. Furthermore, this act removed requirements that a veteran must show diagnosis by a medical examination conducted by a medical officer of the then Veterans Bureau or duly qualified physician within the presumptive period. "This provision alone brought within the purview of the legislation thousands of veterans who [until then] had been unable to connect their disabilities with the service so as to be eligible for compensation and [medical care]."[22]

Between the passage of the World War Veterans Act of 1924 and the act to establish a presumption of service connection for chronic and tropical diseases (P.L. 80-748), several additions were made to the list of presumptive diseases through regulation and executive order. With the enactment of P.L. 80-748 on June 24, 1948, the chronic disease and tropical disease categories were significantly expanded through the codification of presumptive diseases that were previously established by regulation and executive order. Moreover, P.L. 80-748 authorized the VA to add additional chronic diseases to the list. In leading up to the passage of P.L. 80-748, the Administrator of VA asserted that the VA rather than Congress was better suited to decide which disease or disease conditions should be made presumptive:

> It is believed that extreme care should be exercised in augmenting the list of diseases to be afforded the presumption. It is the view of the Veterans' Administration that this can best be accomplished by continuing the existing Veterans Regulation No. 1(a), part I, paragraph I(c), and administrative authority to make the medical and adjudicatory determinations.
>
> Determination governing the selection of diseases to be included under the regulation is essentially one of an involved medical and adjudicatory nature. If a list of diseases is provided by statute it is suggested that the consideration of additions to the present list or subsequent additions to any statutory list would require detailed technical considerations by the Congress which in the opinion of the Veterans' Administration can best be handled administratively. Considering all the facts and circumstances, it is believed that your committee will desire to consider the inadvisability of introducing statutory presumptions of service connection for specific diseases.[23]

1950s-1980s

With the passage of the Veterans Benefits Act of 1957 (P.L. 85-56), Congress codified all laws affecting veterans benefits including the existing list of presumptions and expanded this list by incorporating various presumptions of chronic diseases and disease categories that had been established by regulation and were in effect at that time. At the time P.L. 85-56 was enacted on June 17, 1957, there were 40 chronic diseases or disease categories and 17 tropical diseases that were presumptively service-connected. The 1960s did not see any significant legislative or regulatory changes affecting presumptions of service connection.

The next major legislative change occurred with the enactment of P.L. 91-376 in August 1970. This law established a presumption of service connection for seven categories of diseases and conditions for any veteran held as a prisoner of war (POW) in World War II, the Korean conflict, or the Vietnam War, and who suffered from dietary deficiencies, forced labor, or inhumane treatment in violation of the terms of the Geneva Conventions of July 27, 1929, and August 12, 1949.

It should be noted that up until the late 1970's all the statutory presumptions specified a time period in which a disease or illness needed to have manifested itself. Typically this period was up to one year after separation from active service.

In August 1981, Congress passed the Former Prisoner of War Benefits Act of 1981 (P.L. 97-37). This act, among other things, modified the list of statutory presumptions associated with POW status and also changed the presumptive period for eligibility. The Veterans' Compensation and Program Improvements Amendments of 1984 (P.L. 98-223); the Veterans'

Benefits Improvements and Health Care Authorization Act of 1986 (P.L. 99-576); and the Veterans' Benefits and Services Act of 1988 (P.L. 100-322) expanded the list of diseases in former POWs for which a presumption of service connection was made. Prior to the passage of the Veterans' Health Care, Training and Small Business Loan Act of 1981 (P.L. 97-72), veterans who complained of Agent Orange-related illnesses were at the lowest priority for treatment at VA medical facilities because these conditions were not considered service-connected. P.L. 97-72 elevated Vietnam veterans' priority status for health care at VA facilities by recognizing a veteran's own report of exposure as sufficient proof to receive medical care unless there was evidence to the contrary.

After taking into consideration the "apprehension and concern among some Vietnam veterans and their families…to the alleged ill-health effects among some Vietnam veterans…to exposure to the dioxin in Agent Orange,"[24] Congress passed the Veterans' Dioxin and Radiation Exposure Compensation Standards Act of 1984 (P.L. 98-542). The act required the VA to develop regulations for disability compensation for Vietnam veterans exposed to Agent Orange. Veterans seeking compensation for a condition they thought to be related to herbicide exposure had to provide proof of a service connection that established the link between the exposure and the disease onset. P.L. 98-542 also authorized disability compensation payments to Vietnam veterans for the skin condition chloracne, which was linked to Agent Orange exposure in numerous epidemiologic studies.[25] This law also established a program to provide disability compensation to radiation-exposed veterans who participated in the U.S. atmospheric atomic tests or in the U.S. occupation of Hiroshima and Nagasaki, Japan. Similar to veterans exposed to Agent Orange, these so-called atomic veterans also had to provide evidence of exposure to receive compensation.

In response to atomic veterans' complaints about the difficulty of getting compensation under P.L. 98-542, Congress in 1988 enacted the Radiation-Exposed Veterans' Compensation Act (P.L. 100-321) which established a presumption of a service connection for 13 specified types of cancer. That list was subsequently expanded, first by legislation, later through the VA administrative action, to 21 cancers.[26]

1990s-2000

In 1991, the Agent Orange Act (P.L. 102-4) established for the first time a presumption of service connection for diseases associated with herbicide exposure (discussed in greater detail below). Under the Agent Orange Act, veterans seeking disability compensation for diseases they thought to be associated with herbicides were no longer required to provide proof of exposure. P.L. 102-4 authorized the VA to contract with the IOM to conduct a scientific review of the evidence linking certain medical conditions to herbicide exposure. According to an article published in 2005 in the *Journal of Law and Policy*: "The [IOM] process has become an essential step in ensuring that new service connection presumptions command scientific credibility."[27]

The Veterans' Radiation Exposure Amendments of 1992 (P.L. 102-578) amended P.L. 100-321 by adding two more cancers to the presumptive list. This expansion of the list of cancers was based on the "Biological Effects of Ionizing Radiation V" (BEIR V) report by the National Academy of Sciences.[28] The law also repealed the disability compensation requirement that diseases suffered by radiation-exposed veterans must be manifested within 40 years of exposure.

During the mid-1990's, Congress examined disability compensation issues pertaining to Persian Gulf War[29] veterans. In November 1994, Congress enacted the Persian Gulf War Veterans' Benefits Act (P.L. 103-446), allowing the VA to pay compensation benefits to veterans for Gulf War–related disabilities caused by undiagnosed illnesses. This act also codified the VA's regulatory presumptions based on exposure to herbicides for these types of cancer: Hodgkin's disease, multiple myeloma, and respiratory cancers; and porphyria cutanea tarda, a metabolic disease (must occur within one year of exposure).

In 1998, Congress enacted the Persian Gulf War Veterans Act of 1998 (P.L. 105-277), and the Veterans Programs Enhancement Act of 1998 (P.L. 105-368). Similar to the Agent Orange presumptive program, these laws mandated regular and thorough reviews of the scientific and medical literature relevant to the health of Gulf War veterans by the IOM.

The Veterans Education and Benefits Expansion Act of 2001 (P.L. 107-103) expanded the definition of "qualifying chronic disability" to include a "medically unexplained chronic multisymptom illness (such as chronic fatigue syndrome, fibromyalgia, and irritable bowel syndrome) that is defined by a cluster of signs or symptoms."[30] Furthermore, the Veterans Benefits Act of 2003 (P.L. 108-183) provided a presumption of service connection for cold weather injuries, traumatic arthritis, and certain psychiatric disabilities in former POWs, without regard to length of interment. The Veterans' Housing Opportunity and Benefits Improvement Act of 2006 (P.L. 109-233) added atherosclerotic heart disease or hypertensive vascular disease (including hypertensive heart disease) and their complications (including myocardial infarction, congestive heart failure and arrhythmia) and stroke and its complications to the list of diseases presumed to be service-connected in former POWs.

With passage of the National Defense Authorization Act, FY2008 (P.L. 110-181), Congress established a presumption of service connection for purposes of VA medical care for any veteran of the Persian Gulf War who develops an active mental illness (other than psychosis) if such veteran develops such disability: (1) within two years after discharge or release from the active military, naval, or air service; and (2) before the end of the two-year period beginning on the last day of the Persian Gulf War.

On October 10, 2008, the Veterans' Benefits Improvement Act of 2008 (P.L. 110-389) was enacted. Section 106 of this law established a presumption of service connection for osteoporosis for those veterans that the VA determines to have post-traumatic stress disorder (PTSD). It should be noted that presumptive illnesses for POWs fall into two lists.[31] The first list requires no minimum internment period and includes diseases associated with mental trauma and acute physical trauma. Therefore, such diseases are presumptively service-connected for POWs even with a single day of captivity. The second list requires a minimum 30-day internment period, and includes diseases associated with nutritional deficiencies such as osteoporosis. Section 106 of P.L. 110-389 provides a presumptive service connection for osteoporosis for those veterans with PTSD without the 30-day minimum internment requirement.[32]

ESTABLISHMENT OF AGENT ORANGE PRESUMPTIONS

Thirty-five years after the American military presence in Vietnam[33] ended, the controversy surrounding Agent Orange and its possible association with various illnesses of

Vietnam veterans continues unabated.[34] In general, no other presumption of service connection has had so many congressional hearings, or has been so extensively studied and debated as has establishment of presumption of service connection for diseases associated with exposure to Agent Orange. Therefore, this section provides a brief legislative history leading up to the passage of the Agent Orange Act in 1991 (P.L. 102-4). It is followed by a discussion of the Agent Orange Act of 1991.

Historical Context: 1977-1991

The dense jungles of South Vietnam allowed Communist troops to engage in guerrilla warfare during the Vietnam war.[35] On December 4, 1961, President Kennedy authorized the Secretary of Defense to test the military effectiveness of defoliation.[36] This defoliation program in Vietnam was called "Operation Ranch Hand." The first major large-scale spraying operation, to clear enemy infiltration routes, began over the mangrove forests in the Ca Mau peninsula in the southernmost region of the Mekong Delta in September 1962.[37] From 1962 to 1971, the U.S. Air Force sprayed nearly 19 million gallons of herbicides in Vietnam, of which at least 11 million gallons were Agent Orange—making it the most widely used herbicide in the war.[38]

In 1977, Congress first became aware of a possible link between disabilities in Vietnam veterans and exposure to Agent Orange when a VA employee charged that Agent Orange had caused a wide variety of disabling conditions and diseases.[39] Since that time Vietnam veterans have attributed various illnesses to Agent Orange exposure, including skin conditions, cancers, chronic diseases, birth defects in children, and numerous other ailments. Since the late 1970s, veterans have urged the VA to provide medical treatment for these disorders and many have filed for disability compensation. Initially, the Department of Defense (DOD) maintained that only a limited number of U.S. military personnel could be positively identified as having been exposed to Agent Orange in South Vietnam (i.e., the crews of aircraft that were used to spray herbicides). However, following the publication of a 1979 General Accounting Office (GAO) report documenting ground troop exposure, DOD acknowledged that ground troops were also exposed to Agent Orange.[40] Likewise, the VA consistently took the position that since the long-term exposure to Agent Orange was unclear, and because of scientific uncertainty of the evidence linking Agent Orange to specific illnesses, it could not compensate veterans who alleged that exposure to Agent Orange had caused their diseases. In testifying before the House Committee on Veterans' Affairs, the then Administrator of Veterans Affairs stated:

> Unless or until some such latent effects of Agent Orange or its derivative components are scientifically documented there are intrinsic limitations to VA's authority to allow these [Agent Orange] claims under current law. Though I cannot emphasize enough our policy to resolve reasonable doubt as to service incurrence of disabilities in favor of claimants, there is currently no medical basis upon which adverse health effects of late-post-exposure onset can be reasonably tied to Agent Orange.[41]

In general, in the early days of the Agent Orange controversy issues fell into three categories:

1. compensation for disabilities possibly related to exposure;
2. answers to questions about the health effects of exposure to Agent Orange; and
3. access to health care for diseases that might be related to the exposure.[42]

From 1979 onward, Congress addressed these issues through various legislative measures. In 1979, in response to concerns expressed regarding possible delayed adverse health effects as a result of exposure to Agent Orange, Congress enacted the Veterans Health Programs Extension and Improvement Act of 1979 (P.L. 96-151). It mandated the VA to conduct an epidemiological study of the possible health effects in veterans who served in Vietnam of exposure to dioxin as found in herbicides including Agent Orange. The scope of that study was expanded by section 401 of the Veterans' Health Care, Training and Small Business Loan Act of 1981 (P.L. 97-72), which authorized the inclusion of an evaluation of the impact on the health of Vietnam veterans of exposure to other environmental factors which may have occurred in Vietnam. In 1983, the VA transferred to Centers for Disease Control and Prevention (CDC) the responsibility for this entire study.[43] Moreover, P.L. 97-72 authorized the Department to provide certain health-care services to any veteran of the Vietnam era who while serving in Vietnam may have been exposed to dioxin or to a toxic substance in a herbicide or defoliant used for military purposes.[44] P.L. 97-72 allowed veterans to receive health care even if there was insufficient medical evidence to conclude that their medical condition was associated with exposure to Agent Orange. However, the VA did not acknowledge a link between Agent Orange and those diseases, with the exception of chloracne.[45]

According to the *VA's Analysis of Presumptions of Service Connection:*

> Congress' rationale in enacting this legislation, as it related to [Agent Orange] dioxin, was that: [U]ntil the scientific community [is] able to make a determination as to the possible cause and effect relationship of the toxic herbicides utilized as defoliants in the Republic of Vietnam during the Vietnam conflict, the Veterans' Administration should do everything possible to provide the [health] care to such veterans. When a doubt exists, the doubt should be resolved in favor of the veteran.[46]

In addition to the scientific study mandated in P.L. 96-151 and expanded in P.L. 97-72, numerous scientific studies were conducted related to Agent Orange, and the Vietnam experience as a whole, involving the Veterans' Administration, the Environmental Protection Agency (EPA), and the Departments of Health and Human Services, Defense, and Agriculture.

However, the issue of whether to provide disability compensation to veterans exposed to Agent Orange was not taken up by Congress until 1983. In the 98th Congress several measures were introduced[47] that would have created presumptions of service connection for particular diseases and/or directed VA to conduct rulemaking on the subject of presumptions.[48] Several hearings were held in which witnesses testified and provided their views on the proposed measures. One bill, the Vietnam Veterans Agent Orange Relief Act (H.R. 1961) would have allowed for the presumption of service connection for three diseases:

chloracne (a severe form of acne), soft tissue sarcomas (cancers), and porphyria cutanea tarda (disorder characterized by thinning and blistering of the skin in sun-exposed areas). The measure would have also permitted the Department to add other medical conditions through regulations upon determination that Agent Orange may have caused them. H.R. 1961 contained a sunset clause that would have terminated the presumption upon completion of the study mandated by the Veterans Health Programs Extension and Improvement Act of 1979 (P.L. 96-151). Dozens of witnesses testified with widely divergent views on the bill.[49] The then Administrator of the VA opposed the measure stating that

> The compensation program must be attuned to justifiable conclusions about the connection between Agent Orange exposure and disorders possibly arising from that exposure. At the same time we must do our best to avoid taking steps that have the potential for undermining the program's credibility and legitimacy because of inconclusive scientific evidence.... In view of the current state of scientific findings, enactment [of H.R. 1961] would compromise the integrity of the compensation program and engender unfounded fears among Vietnam veterans that lethal illnesses may yet befall them as a result of having answered the duty's call. [50]

On January 30,1984, the House passed H.R. 1961, as amended, to provide for VA disability compensation, a presumption of service connection for the following three diseases: soft tissue sarcoma, porphyria cutanea tarda, and chloracne. As under the original bill, benefits would terminate one year after the CDC epidemiological study, mandated by the Veterans Health Programs Extension and Improvement Act of 1979 (P.L. 96-151), was submitted to Congress. The Senate passed a different version of H.R. 1961 on May 22, 1984. The Senate-passed version did not provide compensation to veterans exposed to Agent Orange. Rather, the Senate bill addressed the process by which the VA handles Agent Orange by establishing rulemaking guidelines to be used by the VA in adjudicating these claims. The Senate bill also provided for judicial review for both the rulemaking process and individual veterans' compensation claims. The final version of H.R. 1961 was enacted into law on October 24, 1984, as the Veterans' Dioxin and Radiation Exposure Compensation Standards Act, (P.L. 98-542).

As stated previously, P.L. 98-542 required the VA to prescribe regulations regarding the determination of service connection of disabilities of veterans who were exposed to herbicides containing dioxin while serving in Vietnam during the Vietnam era. Section 6 of the statute established the Veterans' Advisory Committee on Environmental Hazards and charged the Advisory Committee to provide the VA with evaluations of pertinent scientific studies relating to possible adverse health effects of exposure to dioxin and with recommendations for legislative or administrative action. Section 5(b) of the statute directed VA to issue regulations establishing guidelines ''governing the evaluation of the findings of scientific studies relating to the possible increased risk of adverse health effects of exposure to herbicides containing dioxin or of exposure to ionizing radiation.'' Section 5(b) further provided that the referenced evaluations of scientific studies would be made by the Administrator (now Secretary) of Veterans Affairs after receiving the advice of the Advisory Committee. Finally, section 5(b) provided that, under the prescribed regulations, VA would make determinations as to whether, and in what circumstances, service connection would be granted for particular diseases based on a finding that a disease is associated with exposure to herbicides containing dioxin.

As this section has illustrated, the attitudes and responses of both Congress and the VA evolved over time as more information regarding Agent Orange, exposure to Agent Orange, and the long range health effects became available. Congress initiated hearings to explore the impact of Agent Orange exposure on the Vietnam veterans' population. In the early days of congressional inquiry, the VA was reluctant to recognize a nexus between Agent Orange exposure and certain illnesses in the veteran population. However, this position was modified as more information became available, and as veterans sought compensation for certain illnesses. In attempting to respond to these concerns, Congress directed the VA to conduct a study of possible delayed adverse health effects in 1979 (Veterans Health Programs Extension and Improvement Act of 1979, P.L. 96-151, §307, 93 Stat. 1092, 1097).

In addition to authorizing the VA to conduct a study on the health effects of Agent Orange exposure, Congress in P.L. 97-72 directed the VA to provide priority health care to Vietnam veterans who were suffering from illnesses believed to be caused by exposure to Agent Orange in Vietnam. Congress directed the VA to provide priority healthcare to Agent Orange-exposed Vietnam veterans on an interim basis until the results of the study authorized by P.L. 96-151 became available. In 1984, five years after authorizing the Agent Orange study in P.L. 96-151, Congress enacted legislation requiring the VA to establish guidelines for deciding disability compensation claims brought by Vietnam veterans exposed to Agent Orange. The new law also required the VA to create and consult with a scientific advisory committee on the adverse health effects of dioxin exposure and, for the first time, mandated compensation payments for Vietnam veterans suffering from two diseases, chloracne and porphyria cutanea tarda, for a two-year period.[51]

Agent Orange Act of 1991 (P.L. 102-4)

Agent Orange legislation in the 99th Congress mainly dealt with studies affecting the health of Vietnam veterans rather than compensation issues. The 100th Congress also continued to generally address the same issues raised in previous Congresses, specifically the on-going issue of determining if health problems among Vietnam veterans exposed to Agent Orange can be attributed to their exposure and how to make that determination.

Despite the passage of the Veterans' Dioxin and Radiation Exposure Compensation Standards Act, (P.L. 98-542), there were concerns among Vietnam veterans about the various scientific studies that were being conducted on the human health effects associated with herbicide exposure during Vietnam service. Furthermore, in 1989, in the case of *Nehmer et al. v. United States Veterans' Administration et al.*[52] "the court held that VA had erred in two key ways in carrying out the requirement in P.L. 98-542. First, by utilizing too high a standard for determining if there is a linkage between exposure to Agent Orange and a subsequent manifestation of a disease and, second, by failing to give the benefit of the doubt to veterans in prescribing the standards in the regulations for VA to use in deciding whether to provide service connection for any specific disease."[53] In response to these concerns in 1991, after numerous hearings, Congress enacted the Agent Orange Act of 1991 on February 6, 1991(P.L. 102-4). The law codified presumption of service connection for chloracne, non-Hodgkin's lymphoma, and soft tissue sarcoma (other than osteosarcoma, chondrosarcoma,

Kaposi's sarcoma, or mesothelioma) associated with Agent Orange. This law also transferred the responsibility of reviewing the scientific literature concerning the association between herbicide exposure during Vietnam service and each health outcome suspected to be associated with such exposure from the VA's Advisory Committee on Environmental Hazards to the National Academy of Sciences.

Moreover, P.L. 102-4 established an entirely new process for evaluating the health effects of exposure to herbicides containing dioxin and for establishing presumptions of service connection for diseases associated with such exposure. The Agent Orange Act requires the Secretary of the VA to conduct new rulemaking proceedings to determine which diseases are sufficiently associated with exposure to Agent Orange so that veterans with approved diseases receive a presumption of service connection. The law states that

> (1) Whenever the Secretary determines, on the basis of sound medical and scientific evidence, that a positive association exists between (A) the exposure of humans to an herbicide agent, and (B) the occurrence of a disease in humans, the Secretary shall prescribe regulations providing that a presumption of service connection is warranted for that disease for the purposes of this section.
> (2) In making determinations for the purpose of this subsection, the Secretary shall take into account (A) reports received by the Secretary from the National Academy of Sciences under section 3 of the Agent Orange Act of 1991, and (B) all other sound medical and scientific information and analyses available to the Secretary.
> (3) An association between the occurrence of a disease in humans and exposure to an herbicide agent shall be considered to be positive for the purposes of this section if the credible evidence for the association is equal to or outweighs the credible evidence against the association.[54]

The Agent Orange Act directed the Secretary to enter into an agreement with the National Academy of Sciences to perform the services as required by the act, and under that agreement, the Academy was to "review and summarize the scientific evidence, and assess the strength concerning the association between exposure to [dioxin] ... and each disease suspected to be associated with such exposure." Moreover, the Academy was to submit its first report no later than 18 months after the enactment of the Agent Orange Act, and, thereafter submit "periodic written reports ... at least once every two years (as measured from the date of the first report)." Furthermore, under the Agent Orange Act, when the Secretary received a report from the Academy, he was required to determine within 60 days "whether a presumption of service connection is warranted for each disease covered by the report," and if he determined that a "presumption is warranted," he was required to issue proposed regulations within 60 days setting forth his determination and to issue final regulations within 90 days after proposing them.[55]

Finally, the Agent Orange Act, as originally enacted, set forth a sunset date for the operation of the provisions that required the Secretary to issue regulations designating service-connected diseases in response to the scientists' reports.[56] The sunset date would be 10 years after the first day of the fiscal year in which the Academy transmitted its first report to the Secretary, and as the first report was transmitted on July 27, 1993, the original effective sunset date was September 30, 2002.

In 2001, 10 years after the passage of the Agent Orange Act, Congress enacted the Veterans Education and Benefits Expansion Act of 2001 (P.L. 107-103). This act amended the sunset date and extended the Secretary's authority to issue regulations designating service connected ailments for another 13 years.[57] Since 1994, as required by law, IOM has issued eight reports concerning associations between health outcomes and exposure to Agent Orange. In addition, IOM has issued three special reports concerning Agent Orange and Type 2 diabetes, Agent Orange and acute myelogenous leukemia in offspring of Vietnam veterans, and the length of presumptive period for association between exposure to Agent Orange and respiratory cancer.

In sum, the Agent Orange Act codified presumptions of service connection for chloracne, non-Hodgkin's lymphoma, and soft tissue sarcoma associated with Agent Orange exposure in Vietnam. With respect to the VA's disability claims process, these presumptions helped to streamline the claims process by allowing Vietnam veterans to establish the second element (in-service occurrence or aggravation of disease) and third element (nexus between in-service occurrence/aggravation of disease and current disease) of the prima facie case for disability compensation, in spite of "[the absence] of evidence of such disease during the period of such service."[58] Additionally, the Agent Orange Act established an entirely new process for evaluating the health effects of exposure to dioxin and other chemical compounds in herbicides and for establishing presumptions of service connection for diseases associated with such exposure. Congress, however, expressly provided that such presumptions created by the VA Secretary pursuant to his authority under the Agent Orange Act may be rebutted by the VA with affirmative evidence establishing that (1) the veteran was not exposed to Agent Orange during service; (2) the veteran's current disability was triggered by an "intercurrent injury or disease" suffered after separation from service; or (3) the veteran's current disease was caused by his own "willful misconduct."[59] **Appendix A** provides a list of presumptive disease conditions that have been established by the VA and Congress based on exposure to Agent Orange. The next section provides an overview of the current process for establishing presumptions for Agent Orange related conditions as well as for other emerging environmental exposures in veterans.

CURRENT PROCESS FOR PRESUMPTIVE DISABILITY DECISIONS[60]

The current process for establishing presumptive disability decisions involves four major entities: Congress, the VA, the Institute of Medicine (IOM), and other stakeholders, which include— among others—veterans service organizations (VSOs) (See **Figure 1**). As discussed earlier, from time-to-time, Congress has exercised its power to create presumptive disability decisions through legislation but has also delegated authority to the Secretary of the VA to establish presumptions in certain instances.[61] Some presumptive decisions have been challenged in court, leading to a revision of the statutes governing the administration of disability compensation by the VA. For example, in the Veterans' Dioxin and Radiation Exposure Compensation Standards Act of 1984 ("Dioxin Act"), Congress authorized the Secretary of the VA to determine which diseases warranted a presumption of service connection relating to Agent Orange exposure during the Vietnam war.[62] Pursuant to the Dioxin Act, the Secretary promulgated a regulation, which provided (1) a presumption of Agent Orange exposure for any veteran who served in Vietnam and (2) a presumption that a single disorder—chloracne—would be considered service connected and thus, eligible for disability compensation.[63] Because the Secretary determined that there was no "cause and effect" relationship between Agent Orange exposure and two other diseases, the Secretary declined to provide any other disease (besides chloracne) with a presumption of service connection.[64]

As stated previously, in 1989, a federal district court invalidated this regulation because "...although Congress [pursuant to Dioxin Act] intended the VA to predicate service connection upon a finding of a significant statistical association between dioxin exposure and various diseases, the VA had erroneously required proof that a causal relationship existed."[65]

VA Presumptive Disability Decisions

A presumption established through legislation usually follows a process through which individual constituents seeking redress from a denial of disability benefits from the VA bring their issues to the attention of Congress. VSOs representing a contingent of veterans or, on rare occasions, executive branch agencies have also lobbied Congress to consider certain presumptions. Through a 1921 amendment to the War Risk Insurance Act (P.L. 63-193), Congress also granted the Secretary of the VA authority to establish regulatory presumptions (P.L. 67-47).

Role of the Institute of Medicine (IOM)

As previously noted, the Agent Orange Act of 1991 established a new process for evaluating the health effects of exposure to herbicides containing dioxin and for establishing presumptions of service connection for diseases associated with such exposure. P.L. 102-4 directed the Secretary to enter into an agreement with the National Academy of Sciences to review and summarize available scientific evidence regarding an association between diseases and exposure to herbicides used in Vietnam. This agreement, in turn, led to a model by which additional studies could be conducted, a model which is still used today. The Institute of Medicine, established in the 1970s as the health arm of the National Academy of Sciences, provides VA with reports that describe the strength of evidence with respect to linkage of agents and specific health concerns. VA uses this evidence and other information in internal decision making to decide whether a presumption will be made.[66] Congress requires the VA to respond after receiving an IOM report with a determination as to whether VA will make a service connection for particular health outcomes on a presumptive basis.

The National Academies convenes panels of its own members and other experts to conduct studies using a systematic process involving open public meetings, the submission of information by outside parties, reviews of the literature, and investigations of committee members and staff. Committee deliberations are closed to the public as well as to study sponsors. Report drafts are subject to an external peer review process overseen by the National Academies.[67]

With respect to studies pertaining to possible presumptions, a new IOM committee is convened. As of 2009, the IOM had completed eight full, biennial Veterans and Agent Orange Reviews and three focused Agent Orange reviews.

Each review examines and characterizes the strength of evidence, such as epidemiologic and toxicological studies, in terms of its association to health outcomes. The first IOM

Veterans and Agent Orange committee characterized the strength of evidence into the following four categories:

1. sufficient evidence of an association;
2. limited/suggestive evidence of an association;
3. inadequate/insufficient evidence to determine whether an association exists; and
4. limited/suggestive evidence of no association.[68]

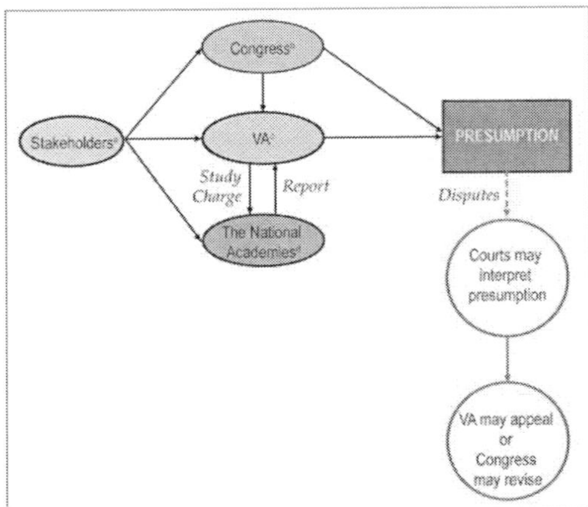

Source: From 'FIGURE S-1' in National Academy of Sciences, Institute of Medicine, *Improving the Presumptive Disability Decision-Making Process for Veterans*, Washington, DC, 2008, p. 11.

Notes:

a. Stakeholders include (but are not limited to) veterans service organizations (VSOs), veterans, advisory groups, federal agencies, and the general public; these stakeholders provide input into the presumptive process by communicating with Congress, VA, and independent organizations (e.g., the National Academies).

b. Congress has created many presumptions itself; in 1921, Congress also empowered the VA Secretary to create regulatory presumptions; on several occasions in the past, Congress has directed VA to contract with an independent organization (e.g., the National Academies) to conduct studies and then use the organization's report in its deliberations of granting or not granting regulatory presumptions.

c. VA can establish regulatory presumptions; VA sometimes contracts with the National Academies to conduct studies and uses the organization's report in its deliberations of granting or not granting regulatory presumptions.

d. The National Academies (Institute of Medicine and National Research Council) submit reports to VA based on requests and study charges from VA.

Figure 1. Roles of the Participants Involved in the Presumptive Disability Decision-Making Process for Veterans.

VA Presumptive Disability Deliberation Process

The VA has followed a general internal review process for evaluating the study findings from IOM and making recommendations to the Secretary of the VA on whether a specific condition(s) should be granted presumptive status. This process includes an initial review by a working group, a subsequent review by a high-level task force, and a final review by the VA Secretary.

Following the submission of the study findings from IOM, a working group is convened, consisting of representatives from several different parts of the VA. Based on the IOM study findings, review of other relevant academic literature, and possible input from various stakeholders, the working group determines whether there is sufficient scientific evidence to support giving any disease(s) special consideration with respect to disability presumptions. Following deliberations, the working group generates a report, which makes recommendations to an internal VA Task Force based on pre-established legal standards by which the VA Secretary's final decision is bound.

The VA internal review Task Force typically consists of high-level officials who report directly to the Secretary. The Task Force reviews the findings of the Working Group and may provide a separate, but similar, report to the VA Secretary based on the Working Group's recommendations. If the Task Force recommends that a new disability presumption be established, and the Secretary concurs, the Veterans Benefits Administration (VBA) will submit a cost estimate and draft regulations for the presumption(s) to the Office of Management and Budget (OMB) for review. If approved by OMB, the proposed rule is then published in the Federal Register. After the allotted period for public comment, the VBA will then prepare a final rule to be submitted to the Federal Register. A more detailed discussion of VA's review of IOM's findings is provided in **Appendix B**.

REPRESENTATIVES AT EACH TIER OF VA'S INTERNAL REVIEW OF IOM REPORTS

Tier 1: Working Group Representatives[69]

- Veterans Health Administration (VHA) Office of Public Health and Environmental Hazards (OPHEH)
- Veterans Benefits Administration (VBA)—Compensation and Pension Service (C&P Service)
- Office of the General Counsel (OGC)—Professional Staff Group II
- VHA personnel with specialized medical training or experience
- Outside technical experts such as National Institutes of Health (NIH), Centers for Disease Control and Prevention (CDC), and Environmental Protection Agency (EPA), as needed

Tier 2: Task Force Representatives[70]

- Under Secretary for Health
- Under Secretary for Benefits
- General Counsel
- Assistant Secretary for Policy and Planning
- Other experts (CDC, EPA, as appropriate)

Tier 3: The VA Secretary

Source: Adapted from "Box 3-1" in National Academy of Sciences, Institute of Medicine, *Improving the Presumptive Disability Decision-Making Process for Veterans*, Washington, DC, 2008, p.59.

Presumptive Disability Decisions: Challenges and Concerns

As part of its 2008 study of the current presumptive disability decision making process, IOM conducted several open meetings to solicit input from stakeholders on their experience with the presumption process. A general concern expressed by some stakeholders was that the IOM is not charged with giving guidance on non-military exposures or alternate causes of certain diseases.[71]

Challenges Facing IOM Presumptive Disability Committees

As noted in the 2008 IOM study on the presumptive disability decision making process studying the evidence base relevant to establishing service connection face the following challenges:

- few directly applicable epidemiologic studies;
- no contemporaneous exposure measurements;
- uncertainty about which veterans were exposed to which agents;
- multiple, possibly synergistic exposures;
- possible long latency for health effects from some agents; and
- significant confounders.[72]

The practice of categorizing the strength of evidence is intended to assist the VA in making evidence-based decisions. However, limitations in evidence inhibits the ability of IOM committees to establish causal relationships between military exposures and long-term health effects. IOM therefore has made recommendations to DOD and VA intended to improve the evidence on exposures and health status of veterans.[73]

Concerns Expressed by Presumptive Disability Policy Makers

The narrowed scope of IOM research also presents a dilemma for VA policy makers whose interpretation of study results are used to help determine which condition(s), if any, are given presumptive status in evaluating disability benefits. For example, past IOM committees have not been asked to evaluate the effects that certain exposures–common in nonmilitary settings–may have on the health of veterans. Additionally, potential exposures may vary for individual veterans depending upon where the veteran was deployed in proximity to hazardous conditions. VA does not collect data on the exposure risk of individual veterans; therefore, IOM specifically reports that the VA is "…hindered by not having exposure data for individuals."[74] The combination of these factors makes it difficult to establish a direct cause-and-effect relationship between military exposures and the specific health condition(s). Indeed, based on current statute, the VA is not required to consider evidence on exposure magnitude or duration and all exposures are given equal weight when determining health effects.[75]

Policy Options

This section briefly discusses two major policy options for the current process to establish presumptions related to exposure to Agent Orange: (1) retain the process; or (2) revise the process. Any change to the current process, which is authorized in statute, would require legislation.

Retain the Current Process

If the current process were retained, the likelihood increases that conditions that are associated with age and lifestyle—as opposed to chemical exposure—may become presumptive.

In addition, continuing the current system may also place veterans of more recent conflicts including Gulf War I, Operation Iraqi Freedom (OIF) and Operation Enduring Freedom (OEF) in a less favorable position for presumptive conditions than Vietnam veterans. Unlike the situation with Vietnam veterans, in which the IOM is able to evaluate a substantial body of scientific literature on the possible association between various diseases of interest and specific type of exposure (i.e. herbicides), the plight of veterans who served in the Gulf region is far more challenging. Not only are there concerns about dozens of different and unrelated environmental hazards (some not under the control of U.S. Armed Forces), but many of the Gulf War era veterans have complex multi-symptomatic conditions that have not been fully diagnosed:

> The VA has had difficulty applying the [IOM] findings to Gulf War veterans because nearly all of the reviewed Gulf War-related hazards represent common, well-characterized occupational exposures that are experienced by virtually all Americans. It may come as a surprise to learn that military environmental exposures generally closely mirror the environmental exposures experienced by all Americans.[76]

Refine the Current Disability Presumption Process

Refinement of the current disability presumptions process would require establishing criteria that convert the current VA process to a more formalized and transparent method of determining what service-connected conditions will be given presumptive status. Specific improvements might include (1) the creation of panels, independent of the VA, to review illnesses to be considered for presumptions and make recommendations the VA Secretary; (2) using *causation*, rather than a positive *association* as the standard for establishing presumptions; and (3) imposing time limits on veterans' presumption claims.

Independent Review of Proposed Presumptions

The use of independent advisory panels prior to conducting IOM-commissioned studies and during deliberations to determine which condition(s) will be recommended for presumption to the VA Secretary has been proposed as one option to increase transparency in the presumptive disability process.

Currently, the VA Secretary initiates deliberations for presumptive disabilities based primarily on issues raised by VSOs, Congress, or other stakeholders representing veterans in the presumption process. To ensure transparency in how the decision to study certain condition(s) is developed, an advisory committee consisting of an independent panel of experts could convene annually to review proposed conditions and nominate condition(s) for further study based on available scientific evidence that illustrates a connection between a certain exposure and a specific health outcome. Public input could also be incorporated into the deliberation process. The advisory committee, rather than the VA, could then charge IOM, or another independent research-based entity, with conducting a study of the condition(s) that have been fully vetted.

Following the conclusion of IOM-commissioned studies, the VA follows a general internal review process that includes an initial review by a working group consisting of VA representatives and needed technical experts. A report from the working group is then forwarded to a high-level task force which makes recommendations directly to the VA Secretary. The duties for reviewing the results of IOM studies and making recommendations to the VA Secretary could also be delegated to an independent panel, with deliberations open to the public.

Use Causation as Basis for Presumptions

The Agent Orange Act of 1991 (P.L. 102-4) established the threshold for determining a presumption based only on a positive *association* between herbicide exposure and a health outcome as opposed to using *causation* as the basis. As a result, IOM Agent Orange committees have used a framework based on association (sufficient, limited/suggestive, inadequate/insufficient, and no association) between herbicide exposure and specific health outcomes rather than identifying direct causal mechanisms.

Under current law, a positive association (between dioxin or other compounds in herbicides and a specific condition) exists if the "credible" evidence for an association is equal to or outweighs the "credible" evidence against an association.[77] Also, under law, if a positive association exists, the Secretary is required to issue regulations making the condition presumptive.[78]

As an alternative, following the conclusion of any IOM-commissioned studies and post-study reviews, the VA Secretary could be statutorily restricted to only implementing presumptions for conditions that have a clear and/or direct causal link to military service based on scientific evidence. Conditions where evidence of a service connection does not meet the *causal* threshold, should automatically trigger further research before the Secretary is required to make the condition presumptive. A supplemental study examining the prevalence of the condition among veterans who were deployed to an affected region as compared to an analogous group of veterans who were not deployed could assist in determining whether that condition is more prevalent among the affected veterans than the non-affected veterans. Data and technical experts from other federal agencies such as the National Institutes of Health (NIH), the CDC, and the EPA could assist in conducting this supplemental study. Condition(s) that are determined to have a strong association with certain exposures, coupled with statistical evidence of higher prevalence rates among the affected veterans, could be deemed sufficient for establishing a presumption.

Impose Time Limitations on Presumption Claims

An individual's lifestyle, genetic heritage, and/or the aging process can have an effect on the development of a variety of medical conditions. The influence of these factors is currently not considered in the current presumption process. A health condition related to military service can be expected to manifest within a proximate time period from exposure, and many diseases have multiple risk factors. As time passes, age and lifestyle factors may have a greater influence on the development of a health condition than prior exposure. Using scientific knowledge to impose time limitations on when a condition(s) could be considered "service-connected" may help to reduce the likelihood that extraneous factors—unrelated to military service—influence the determination (or applicability) of presumptions.

APPENDIX A. DISEASE CONDITIONS PRESUMPTIVELY SERVICE-CONNECTED

Table A-1. Presumptive Service-Connected Diseases Based on Exposure to Agent Orange, 1985-2010

Presumptive Disease	Legislation or Regulation Establishing Presumption	Date Established
Chloracne (a severe form of acne).	Adjudication of Claims Based on Exposure to Dioxin or Ionizing Radiation. Final rules. *Federal Register*, 50(165):34452- 34461.	August 26, 1985
Non-Hodgkin's lymphoma (large group of cancers of lymphocytes-white blood cells).	Claims Based on Service in Vietnam. Final regulation. *Federal Register*, 55(208):43123- 43125.	October 6, 1990
Soft tissue sarcoma (soft tissue sarcoma is a cancer of soft tissues such as muscles, tendons, and blood vessels). Does not include osteosarcoma, chondrosarcoma, Kaposi's sarcoma, or mesothelioma.	Agent Orange Act of 1991 (P.L. 102-4). Codified Chloracne and Non-Hodgkin's lymphoma previously established by regulation and added Soft tissue sarcoma to the list of presumptive conditions.	February 6, 1991
Soft-tissue sarcoma including the following: Adult fibrosarcoma; Dermatofibrosarcoma protuberans; Malignant fibrous histiocytoma; Liposarcoma; Leiomyosarcoma; Epithelioid leiomyosarcoma (malignant leiomyoblastoma); Rhabdomyosarcoma; Ectomesenchymoma; Angiosarcoma (hemangiosarcoma and lymphangiosarcoma); Proliferating (systemic) angioendotheliomatosis; Malignant glomus tumor; Malignant hemangiopericytoma; Synovial sarcoma (malignant synovioma); Malignant giant cell tumor of tendon sheath; Malignant schwannoma, including malignant schwannoma with rhabdomyoblastic differentiation (malignant Triton tumor); glandular and epithelioid malignant schwannomas; Malignant mesenchymoma; Malignant granular cell tumor; Alveolar soft part sarcoma; Epithelioid sarcoma; and Clear cell sarcoma of tendons and aponeuroses.	Claims Based on Exposure to Herbicides Containing Dioxin (Soft-Tissue Sarcomas) Final regulation. *FederalRegister*, 56(199):51651-51653. It should be noted that these regulations were published to implement provisions of P.L. 98-542, which required that determinations as to whether conditions are related to dioxin exposure be made after receiving the advice of the Veterans Advisory Committee on Environmental Hazards (VACEH) based on its reviews of scientific and medical studies.	October 15, 1991
Added the following to the list of soft-tissue sarcomas: Extraskeletal Ewing's sarcoma	Diseases Associated With Service in the Republic of Vietnam. Final rule, *Federal Register*, 58(95):29107- 29109	May 19, 1993

Table A-1. (Continued)

Presumptive Disease	Legislation or Regulation Establishing Presumption	Date Established
Congenital and infantile fibrosarcoma Malignant ganglioneuroma		
Hodgkin's disease (is a type of lymphoma. Lymphoma is cancer of lymph tissue found in the lymph nodes, spleen, liver, and bone marrow). Porphyria cutanea tarda (disorder characterized by thinning and blistering of the skin in sun-exposed areas)	Disease Associated With Exposure to Certain Herbicide Agents. Final rule. *Federal Register*, 59(23):5106-5107.	February 3, 1994
Multiple myeloma (Multiple myeloma is a cancer that begins in plasma cells, a type of white blood cell). Respiratory cancers: Bronchus Larynx Lung Trachea	Disease Associated With Exposure to Certain Herbicide Agents (Multiple Myeloma and Respiratory Cancers) Final rule. *Federal Register*, 59(110):29723-29724.	June 9, 1994
Hodgkin's disease Multiple myeloma Porphyria cutanea tarda Respiratory cancers: Bronchus Larynx Lung Trachea	Persian Gulf War Veterans' Benefits Act of 1994 (P.L. 103-446). This law codified the diseases that were established by regulation since the enactment of the Agent Orange Act of (P.L. 102-4).	November 2, 1994
Prostate cancer Acute and subacute peripheral neuropathy	Diseases Associated With Exposure to Certain Herbicide Agents (Prostate Cancer and Acute and Subacute Peripheral Neuropathy). Final rule. *Federal Register*, 61(217):57586-57589.	November 7, 1996
Type 2 Diabetes (Type 2 diabetes" is also referred to as "Type II diabetes mellitus" or "adult-onset diabetes").	Disease Associated With Exposure to Certain Herbicide Agents: Type 2 Diabetes. Final rule. *Federal Register*, 66(89):23166-23169.	May 8, 2001
Diabetes mellitus (Type 2).	Veterans Education and Benefits Expansion Act of 2001 (P.L. 107-	December

Presumptive Disease	Legislation or Regulation Establishing Presumption	Date Established
	103) codified Type 2 Diabetes that was established by regulation.	27, 2001
Chronic lymphocytic leukemia (is cancer of a type of white blood cells called lymphocytes).	Disease Associated With Exposure to Certain Herbicide Agents: Chronic Lymphocytic Leukemia. Final rule. *Federal Register*, 68(200):59540- 59542.	October 16, 2003
AL amyloidosis (Amyloidosis occurs when abnormal proteins build up and form deposits. The deposits can collect in organs such as the kidney and heart).	Presumptive Service Connection for Disease Associated With Exposure to Certain Herbicide Agents: AL Amyloidosis. Final Rule. *Federal Register* 74(87):21258-21260.	May 7, 2009
Hairy cell leukemia and other chronic B-cell leukemias (rare cancer of the blood. It affects B cells, a type of white blood cell (lymphocyte)). Parkinson's disease (Parkinson's disease is a disorder that affects nerve cells, or neurons, in a part of the brain that controls muscle movement). Ischemic heart disease ("an inadequate supply of blood and oxygen to a portion of the myocardium; it typically occurs when there is an imbalance between myocardial oxygen supply and demand").	Diseases Associated With Exposure to Certain Herbicide Agents (Hairy Cell Leukemia and Other Chronic B-Cell Leukemias, Parkinson's Disease and Ischemic Heart Disease). Final rule. *ederal Register* 75(168):53202-53216.	August 31, 2010

Source: Table prepared by the Congressional Research Service based on Appendix F of in National Academy of Sciences, Institute of Medicine, *Improving the Presumptive Disability Decision-Making Process for Veterans*, Washington, DC, 2008, pp. F2-F43 and *Federal Register* notices.

Notes: Definitions and/or description of diseases obtained from MedlinePlus of the National Institutes of Health http://www.nlm.nih. gov/medlineplus/ and from *Federal Register* notices accompanying the establishment of presumptive diseases.

Appendix B. Summary of VA's Review of IOM Reports[79]

The VA has not adopted formal procedures governing its internal review of IOM reports. However, practice has been it involves a three-tiered review. In the first tier, a "Working Group" of VA employees from different operational elements of the VA reviews the IOM report and any other relevant evidence and prepares a summary of its assessment and a statement of recommendations or options. This summary is intended for the benefit of a "Task Force" composed of high-level VA officials. In the second tier, the Task Force, based on the Working Group's input, provides recommendations to the Secretary, usually in the form of a separate written report. In the third tier, the Secretary determines, based on the Task Force's input, whether a presumption of service connection is warranted for any disease.

VA Working Group

The Working Group ordinarily consists of members of the Office of Public Health and Environmental Hazards (OPHEH) of the Veterans Health Administration (VHA), the Compensation and Pension Service (C&P Service) of the Veterans Benefits Administration (VBA), and representatives from the Office of the General Counsel (OGC). Additionally, the Working Group often includes other VHA personnel with specialized medical training or experience concerning a health issue implicated by a particular IOM report. Members are assigned to the Working Group by supervisory personnel within VHA, VBA, and OGC. The Working Group convenes after receiving the briefing from the IOM committee. Prior to the meeting, VHA personnel seek to identify, based on the IOM report and the committee briefing, the diseases that may warrant special consideration because the IOM's findings with respect to those diseases appear to be potentially significant. At the initial Working Group meeting, VHA provides the Working Group members with additional information concerning those diseases, including copies of any significant scientific studies identified in the IOM report and other information concerning matters such as the course of the disease, known causes or risk factors, related conditions or health effects, latency periods (if any), and any other known relevant information. OGC representative briefs the Working Group on the legal standard governing the Secretary's decision. Members of the Working Group discuss whether any of the IOM's findings appear to be potentially significant, in that they might warrant a presumption of service connection for a particular disease or diseases, and the strength of the scientific evidence with respect to such diseases. The Working Group will attempt to reach consensus as to whether the scientific evidence appears to warrant a presumption of service connection for any diseases under the applicable legal standard. If the Working Group reaches agreement that a presumption is or is not warranted on the basis of the scientific evidence and the legal standard, it will agree to put forth a recommendation based on that conclusion. In arriving at such recommendations, the Working Group relies on scientific evidence and the legal standard, and does not consider matters of governmental policy or cost. If the Working Group concludes that the scientific evidence and legal standard do not provide a clear basis for recommending for or against establishing a presumption, but permit a range of options, the Working Group agrees to set forth a range of options for decision by VA policy-making officials. In those circumstances, the Working Group will discuss the factors that preclude a clear recommendation, which may include ambiguity in the governing statutory standard as applied to certain IOM findings, the limited or conditional nature of the IOM's findings with respect to certain diseases, or other factors. The Working Group will discuss the decisional options available to the Secretary and may also discuss the factors that may be relevant to the Secretary's decision among those options. To this extent, the Working Group may discuss the policy considerations that would be relevant to the Secretary's choice among permissible courses of action. Once the Working Group has reached agreement concerning its recommendations or presentation of options, a written report is completed. The Report will contain (1) a summary of the issues to be decided under applicable law and the IOM report, (2) a summary of the findings contained in the IOM report, (3) a summary of the legal standard governing VA's decision, (4) a summary of the Working Group's analysis of the medical evidence in relation to the legal standard, particularly with respect to any potentially significant findings in the IOM report, and (5) a statement of the Working Group's recommendations or of the options identified by the Working Group. The Working Group does not prepare or obtain a cost estimate for the options, although it may provide general information concerning, e.g., the prevalence rates of certain diseases under consideration. If the Working Group report lists a range of options available to the Secretary, it would identify the scientific and legal considerations relevant to the Secretary's choice among those options, and may also identify policy implications associated with various options.

VA Task Force

The Task Force consists of the Under Secretary for Health, the Under Secretary for Benefits, the General Counsel, and the Assistant Secretary for Policy and Planning. There is no established procedure for the Task Force's deliberations. Task Force members receive a copy of the Working Group report and, based on that report, provide advice to the Secretary concerning the Secretary's determination, which may include recommendations based upon the options, if any, outlined by the Working Group. The Task Force often, though not always, provides a separate report to the Secretary.

Secretary

Based on the Task Force's report, the Secretary determines whether or not to establish presumptions for any diseases discussed in the IOM report and directs appropriate action to implement the decision.

End Notes

[1] U.S. Congress, House Committee on Veterans' Affairs, *The Provision of Federal Benefits for Veterans, An Historical Analysis of Major Veterans Legislation, 1862-1954*, committee print, 84th Cong., 1st sess., December 28, 1955, H.Prt. No. 171, p. 2.

[2] Department of Veterans Affairs, *Veterans Benefits Administration: An Organizational History: 1776-1994*, Washington, DC, November 1995, p. 6. Although the Continental Congress passed resolutions promising

benefits, it lacked the authority and resources to implement these benefit laws, and left this task to individual states.

[3] Currently, there is no statutory definition for the Global War on Terrorism (GWOT). Since the September 11, 2001, terrorist attacks, the Department of Defense (DOD) has been engaged in domestic and overseas military operations. These operations include Operation Noble Eagle aimed at defending the United States homeland against terrorist attacks; Operation Enduring Freedom (OEF) that takes place principally in and around Afghanistan, but also covers additional operations in the Horn of Africa, the Philippines, and elsewhere; and Operation Iraqi Freedom (OIF) that focused principally on Iraq. All these operations have been collectively known as " GWOT." (U.S. Government Accountability Office, *Global War On Terrorism*, GAO-09-302, March 17, 2009, p. 1). It should be noted that on September 1, 2010, OIF was named Operation New Dawn coinciding with the change of mission for U.S. forces in Iraq.

[4] Veterans Benefits Disability Commission, *Honoring the Call to Duty: Veterans' Disability Benefits in the 21st Century*, Washington, DC, October 3, 2007, p. 444.

[5] Department of Veterans Affairs (VA), "Analysis of Presumptions of Service Connection," a report to the Senate Committee on Veterans' Affairs, December 23, 1993.

[6] The Veterans' Disability Benefits Commission was established by the National Defense Authorization Act of 2004 (P.L. 108-136), and was charged with providing a "comprehensive evaluation and assessment of the benefits provided under the laws of the United States to compensate veterans and their survivors for disability or death attributable to military service."

[7] National Academy of Sciences, Institute of Medicine, *Improving the Presumptive Disability Decision-Making Process for Veterans*, Washington, DC, 2008, http://www.nap.edu/ catalog/11908.html.

[8] Between 1962 and 1971, the U.S. Air Force sprayed approximately 107 million pounds of herbicides in South Vietnam for the purpose of defoliation and crop destruction. The herbicides sprayed during the Vietnam era contained mixtures of 2,4-dichlorophenoxyacetic acid (2,4-D), 2,4,5-trichlorophenoxyacetic acid (2,4,5-T), picloram, and cacodylic acid. The most extensively used defoliant compound, a 50:50 combination of 2,4-D and 2,4,5-T, came to be known as "Agent Orange" because of the orange-colored band placed on each chemical storage container (National Academy of Sciences, Institute of Medicine, *Veterans and Agent Orange: Health Effects of Herbicides Used in Vietnam*, Washington , DC, 1994, p. 27).

[9] National Academy of Sciences, Institute of Medicine, *Improving the Presumptive Disability Decision-Making Process for Veterans*, Washington, DC, 2008, p. 342.

[10] 38 U.S.C. §§ 1110, 1131. These provisions deal with the basic entitlement for disability compensation.

[11] For more information see CRS Report RL33323, *Veterans Affairs: Benefits for Service-Connected Disabilities*, by Douglas Reid Weimer.

[12] The term "service-connected" means, with respect to disability or death, that such disability was incurred or aggravated, or that the death resulted from a disability incurred or aggravated, in line of duty in the active military, naval, or air service (38 U.S.C. § 101).

[13] 38 C.F.R. § 3.303.

[14] 38 C.F.R. § 3.306.

[15] 38 C.F.R. § 3.310.

[16] 38 C.F.R. § 1151.

[17] 38 C.F.R. § 3.307.

[18] 38 U.S.C. § 501(a)(1).

[19] Department of Veterans Affairs (VA), "Analysis of Presumptions of Service Connection, " a report to the Senate Committee on Veterans' Affairs, December 23, 1993, p. i.

[20] U.S. Congress, House Committee on Veterans' Affairs, *The Provision of Federal Benefits for Veterans, An Historical Analysis of Major Veterans Legislation, 1862-1954,* committee print, 84th Cong., 1st sess., H. Prt. No 171, December 28, 1955 (Washington: GPO, 1955), p. 21.

[21] Department of Veterans Affairs (VA), "Analysis of Presumptions of Service Connection," a report to the Senate Committee on Veterans' Affairs, December 23, 1993, p. 10.

[22] U.S. Congress, House Committee on Veterans' Affairs, The Provision of Federal Benefits for Veterans, An Historical Analysis of Major Veterans Legislation, 1862-1954, committee print, 84th Cong., 1st sess., House Committee Print No 171, December 28, 1955 (Washington: GPO, 1955), p. 23.

[23] U.S. Congress, Senate Committee on Finance, *Veterans Chronic and Tropical Diseases–Presumption of Service Connection*, report to accompany H.R. 3889, 80th Cong., June 7, 1948.

[24] U.S. Congress, House Committee on Veterans' Affairs, Veterans' Dioxin and Radiation Exposure Compensation Standards Act. Report to Accompany H.R. 1961, 98th Congress, 2nd sess., H.Rept. 98-592.

[25] National Academy of Sciences, Institute of Medicine, *Veterans and Agent Orange: Health Effects of Herbicides Used in Vietnam*, Washington , DC, 1994, p. 678.

[26] For further information, see CRS Report RL33927, *Selected Federal Compensation Programs for Physical Injury or Death*, coordinated by Sarah A. Lister and C. Stephen Redhead.

[27] Mark Brown, "The Role of Science in Department of Veterans Affairs Disability Compensation Policies for Environmental and Occupational Illnesses and Injuries," *Journal of Law and Policy*, vol-13, (2005).

[28] Committee on the Biological Effects of Ionizing Radiation (BEIR), National Research Council, is part of the National Academy of Sciences.

[29] The term "Persian Gulf War" means the period beginning on August 2, 1990, and ending on the date thereafter prescribed by Presidential proclamation or by law (38 U.S.C. §101).

[30] Subsection 202 (a) of the Veterans Education and Benefits Expansion Act of 2001 (P.L. 107-103), December 27, 2001.

[31] 38 U.S.C. §1112(b); 38 C.F.R. §3.309(c).

[32] Department of Veterans Affairs, "Presumption of Service Connection for Osteoporosis for Former Prisoners of War," 74 *Federal Register* 44288, August 28, 2009.

[33] The term "Vietnam era" means the following: (1) The period beginning on February 28, 1961, and ending on May 7, 1975, in the case of a veteran who served in the Republic of Vietnam during that period; (2) the period beginning on August 5, 1964, and ending on May 7, 1975, in all other cases (38 U.S.C. § 101).

[34] Kerry Young, "Vietnam's Toxic Legacy Costs," *CQ Weekly*, May 24, 2010, p. 1251; Kerry Young, "Presumptive Spending in VA Gets New Scrutiny," *CQ Weekly*, June 28, 2010, p. 1547; and David Rogers, "The Bill for Agent Orange Comes Due," *Politico*, August 30, 2010 http://www.politico.com/news/stories/0810/41571.html.

[35] Wilbur J. Scott, "Competing Paradigms in the Assessment of Latent Disorders: The Case of Agent Orange," *Social Problems*, vol. 35, no. 2 (April 1988), p. 146.

[36] National Academy of Sciences, Institute of Medicine, *Characterizing Exposure of Veterans to Agent Orange and Other Herbicides Used in Vietnam*, Scientific Considerations Regarding a Request for Proposals for Research, Washington, DC, 2007, p. 16.

[37] Ibid.

[38] The different types of herbicide used by U.S. forces in Vietnam were identified by a code name referring to the color of the band around the 55-gallon drum that contained the chemical. These included Agents Orange, White, Blue, Purple, Pink, and Green. From 1962 to 1965, small quantities of Agents Purple, Pink, and Green were used in the defoliation program (National Academy of Sciences, Institute of Medicine, *Veterans and Agent Orange: Health Effects of Herbicides Used in Vietnam*, Washington, DC, 1994, p. 27).

[39] U.S. Congress, House Committee on Veterans' Affairs, *Agent Orange in Vietnam: A Report on the Mission to Vietnam*, committee print, prepared by the Honorable Don Edwards, member, House Veterans' Affairs Committee, to the Committee on Veterans Affairs, on his visit to Vietnam, 98th Cong., 2nd sess., January 31, 1984 (Washington: GPO, 1984), p. 1. Also see, National Academy of Sciences, Institute of Medicine, *Veterans and Agent Orange: Health Effects of Herbicides Used in Vietnam*, Washington, DC, 1994, p. 33.

[40] U.S. General Accounting Office, *U.S. Ground Troops in South Vietnam Were in Areas Sprayed with Herbicide Orange*, FBCD 80-23, 1979, http://archive.gao.gov/f0302/110930.pdf.

[41] Statement of Max Cleland, Administrator of Veterans' Affairs in U.S. Congress, House Committee on Veterans' Affairs, Subcommittee on Medical Facilities and Benefits, *Oversight Hearing to Receive Testimony on Agent Orange*, 96th Cong., 2nd sess., February 25, 1980 (Washington: GPO, 1980), p. 11.

[42] U.S. Congress, Senate Committee on Veterans' Affairs, *Veterans Agent Orange Exposure and Vietnam Service Benefits Act of 1989*, report to accompany S. 1153, 101st Cong., 1st sess., July 24, 1989, S.Rept. 101-82 (Washington: GPO, 1989), p. 27.

[44] For more information on health care provided to Vietnam era veterans, see CRS Report RL34370, *Veterans Affairs: Health Care and Benefits for Veterans Exposed to Agent Orange*, by Sidath Viranga Panangala and Douglas Reid Weimer.

[45] Wilbur J. Scott, "Competing Paradigms in the Assessment of Latent Disorders: The Case of Agent Orange," *Social Problems*, vol. 35, no. 2 (April 1988), p. 155.

[46] Department of Veterans Affairs (VA), "Analysis of Presumptions of Service Connection" a report to the Senate Committee on Veterans' Affairs, December 23, 1993, p. 65.

[47] S. 374, 98th Cong., 1st Sess. (1983); S. 786, 98th Cong.,1st Sess. (1983); S. 991, 98th Cong., 1st Sess. (1983); H.R.1961, 98th Cong., 1st. Sess. (1983); and S. 1651, 98th Cong., 1st Sess. (1983).

[48] Department of Veterans Affairs (VA), "Analysis of Presumptions of Service Connection" a report to the Senate Committee on Veterans' Affairs, December 23, 1993, p.66.

[49] U.S. Congress, House Committee on Veterans' Affairs, *Agent Orange and Atomic Veterans Relief Act*, report to accompany H.R. 1961, 98th Cong., 2nd sess., January 25, 1984, p. 4.

[50] Ibid, p.16 and p. 20.

[51] Veterans' Dioxin and Radiation Exposure Compensation Standards Act, (P.L. 98-542) As an illustration of the uncertainty surrounding the eventual codification of presumptive Agent Orange disorders, Representative Tom Ridge expressed this concern:

> One of the concerns I have, I guess, is that if we look [for scientific studies] to establish with an absolute degree of medical or scientific certainty the nexus between exposure to Agent Orange and the variety of maladies that may result from that exposure, we may indeed wait 40 or 50 years [to establish presumptive

Agent Orange disorders] in spite of the efforts of the VA, in spite of the efforts of other countries, in spite of all the tests we run.

Scientific Research on the Health of Vietnam Veterans Hearing on H.R. 3486 Before the Subcomm. on Hospitals and Health Care of the H. Comm. on Veterans' Affairs, 100th Cong. 16 (1988) (statement of Representative Thomas J. Ridge, Member, House Subcommittee on Hospitals and Health Care). Similarly, Senator John Kerry noted in written testimony before the subcommittee:

I believe that it is nothing less than wrong on the facts to tell Vietnam veterans that we cannot compensate for diseases which were caused by their exposure to Agent Orange in Vietnam. It is offensive to veterans to tell them that there is not enough "scientific evidence" to justify compensation ... Our legislation [S. 1787] would establish a presumption of service connection for two of these diseases, non-Hodgkins lymphoma and lung cancer. In addition [S. 1787] would ask the National Academy of Sciences to review the evidence of the scientific studies and compile a list of other diseases which are linked to suppression of the immune system, which may be linked to dioxin or Agent Orange exposure. If appropriate, these diseases would be added and a presumption of service connection [would be] created.

Ibid. at 67-71 (written testimony of Senator John Kerry before House Subcommittee on Hospitals and Health Care).

[52] Nehmer v. U.S. Veterans Admin., 712 F.Supp. at 1420, 1423 (N.D. Cal. 1989).

[53] U.S. Congress, Senate Committee on Veterans Affairs, *Veterans' Agent Orange Exposure and Vietnam Service Benefits Act of 1989*, report to accompany S. 1153, 101st Cong., 1st sess., July 24, 1989 (Washington: GPO, 1989), p. 35.

[54] 38 U.S.C. § 1116 (b).

[55] 38 U.S.C. § 1116(c)(1)(A), (c)(2).

[56] 38 U.S.C. § 316(e), 38 U.S.C.A. § 1116(e) (1992).

[57] As a result, the provisions in 38 U.S.C. § 1116(b), (c) and (d) have remained in effect since 1991, and will continue to be effective until September 30, 2015, or until such other time as Congress shall establish, should it enact another extension.

[58] 38 U.S.C. § 1116(a)(1)(B). *See* Darby v. Brown, 10 Vet.App. 243, 246 (CAVC 1997) (where claimant satisfies requirements of 38 U.S.C. § 1116, "the requirements for evidence of both service incurrence and causal nexus are satisfied").

[59] 38 U.S.C. § 1113(a). *See* Darby v. Brown, 10 Vet.App. at 246-247 (*rebutting* presumption of service connection provided by 38 U.S.C. § 1116 and *denying* disability compensation claim pursuant to 38 U.S.C. § 1113(a)).

[60] Major portions of this section were drawn from National Academy of Sciences, Institute of Medicine , *Improving the Presumptive Disability Decision-Making Process for Veterans*, Washington, DC, 2008.

[61] 38 U.S.C. § 501(a).

[62] P.L. 98-542, 98 Stat. 2725 (1984). [63] 38 C.F.R. §§ 3.311a(b), 3.311a(c) (1988).

[64] 38 C.F.R. § 3.311(d) (1988).

[65] Nehmer v. U.S. Dept. of Veterans Affairs, 494 F.3d 846, 850 (9th Cir. 2007) *quoting* Nehmer v. U.S. Veterans Admin., 712 F.Supp. at 1420, 1423 (N.D. Cal. 1989).

[66] National Academy of Sciences, Institute of Medicine, *Improving the Presumptive Disability Decision-Making Process for Veterans*, Washington, DC, 2008, p.2.

[67] For additional information on the National Academies and the committee process see http://national academies.org/.

[68] IOM was additionally contracted to explore possible links between service in the Gulf War I and a host of medical conditions experienced by veterans known collectively as "Gulf War Syndrome." The IOM committees conducting the Gulf War I studies used a similar categorization process that included (1) sufficient evidence of a causal relationship, (2) sufficient evidence of an association, (3) limited/suggestive evidence of an association, (4) inadequate/insufficient evidence to determine whether an association does or does not exist, and (5) limited/suggestive evidence of no association. With minor changes, these categories are still in use today (National Academy of Sciences, Institute of Medicine, *Improving the Presumptive Disability Decision-Making Process for Veterans*, Washington, DC, 2008, pp. 64-65).

[69] The members generally are assigned to the working group by supervisory personnel within VHA, VBA, and OGC. The working group may receive input from outside content experts as well as veterans, Veterans Service Organizations (VSOs), and Congress.

[70] Appointed by the VA Secretary.

[71] National Academy of Sciences, Institute of Medicine, *Improving the Presumptive Disability Decision-Making Process for Veterans*, Washington, DC, 2008, p.61.

[72] Ibid, pp.64-65.

[73] Ibid, p.24.

[74] Ibid, p.61.

[75] Ibid.

[76] Mark Brown, "Role of Science in Department of Veterans Affairs Disability Compensation Policies for Environmental and Occupational Illnesses and Injuries, The Science for Judges IV," Journal of Law and Policy, vol. 13 (2005), pp. 608-609.

[77] 38 U.S.C. § 1116(b)(3).

[78] 38 U.S.C. § 1116(b)(1).

[79] Adapted from Department of Veterans Affairs, Office of the Secretary, *Final Draft Report of Department of Veterans Affairs Gulf War Illness Task Force to the Secretary of Veterans Affairs*, March 29, 2010, pp. 86-87.

In: Veteran Injuries, Disorders and Medical Care Service
Editors: Jessica Michaels and Jesse E. Levine
ISBN: 978-1-62081-302-7

Chapter 3

SUICIDE, PTSD, AND SUBSTANCE USE AMONG OEF/OIF VETERANS USING VA HEALTH CARE: FACTS AND FIGURES*

Erin Bagalman

On May 10, 2011, the Ninth Circuit Court of Appeals ruled against the Department of Veterans Affairs (VA) in a case brought by two nonprofit veterans advocacy groups, Veterans for Common Sense and Veterans United for Truth.[1] The ruling criticized the VA's mental health services, among other things.[2] This has intensified interest in veterans' mental health, already a topic of ongoing concern to Members of Congress and their constituents.

This brief report addresses three relevant topics: suicide, posttraumatic stress disorder (PTSD), and substance use disorders. Using data from the VA, it answers two questions about each topic: (1) How many veterans of Operations Enduring Freedom and Iraqi Freedom (OEF/OIF)[3] are affected? and (2) What is the VA doing, in terms of screening, prevention, and treatment?

OEF/OIF VETERANS USING VA HEALTH CARE

In general, veterans must enroll with the VA in order to receive VA health care services. All enrolled veterans are offered a standard medical benefits package that covers, among other things, mental health care, including substance abuse treatment; additional benefits may be available, based on service-connected disabilities, income, or other factors.[4]

The VA offers OEF/OIF veterans enhanced enrollment eligibility for five years following separation.[5] From FY2002 through FY2010, a total of 1,250,663 OEF/OIF veterans separated from service. Approximately half of them (625,384) used VA health care at some point during that time.[6]

* This is an edited, reformatted and augmented version of the Congressional Research Service Publication, CRS Report for Congress R41921, dated July 18, 2011.

The VA has provided Congressional Research Service (CRS) with data on these veterans. The data include suicide rates (annual through FY2008), prevalence of PTSD (cumulative across years), and prevalence of substance use disorders (cumulative across years).[7]

The VA uses electronic medical records, which include reminders for required screenings. Providers at the VA can also access electronic records for care provided by the Department of Defense (DOD), including mental health assessments conducted prior to separation.[8]

Systematic information regarding veterans who do not use VA health care is not available. Data about OEF/OIF veterans using VA health care should not be extrapolated to the rest of the OEF/OIF veteran population, or to the broader veteran population. Limitations of the VA's data are discussed in **Appendix A**.

SUICIDE

The VA identifies veteran suicides by matching suicides from the National Death Index[9] with the roster of veterans in VA administrative data. **Figure 1** presents annual suicide rates (i.e., not the number of suicides) among male and female OEF/OIF veterans, separately and combined. Rates are presented per 100,000 OEF/OIF veterans enrolled in VA health care; for example, in FY2008, the rate of suicides was 38 per 100,000 OEF/OIF veterans (male and female combined) enrolled in VA health care.[10] The figure represents only completed (i.e., fatal) suicides; it does not include attempted (i.e., nonfatal) suicides. Data limitations are discussed in **Appendix A**.

Suicide Prevention in the VA Health Care System

Department policy requires an annual depression screening for veterans using VA health care. For each veteran identified as at high risk for suicide, a suicide prevention safety plan is developed, and the veteran's medical record is flagged. The VA has established a center of excellence in suicide prevention, and every VA Medical Center is staffed with a suicide prevention coordinator.[11] All veterans, regardless of enrollment, may use the department's suicide hotline (1-800-273-8255, option 1), an online chat service (www.VeteransCrisisLine.net/chat), and an online suicide prevention resource center (www.suicideoutreach.org) maintained jointly with the DOD. Several reports that have evaluated the department's suicide prevention efforts, and offered recommendations, are listed in **Appendix B**.

POSTTRAUMATIC STRESS DISORDER (PTSD)

Posttraumatic stress disorder (PTSD) is a psychological response to a traumatic event; OEF/OIF Veterans Using VA Health Care, however, a history of trauma is not enough to FY2002-FY2010 establish a diagnosis of PTSD. The diagnosis requires a minimum number of symptoms in each of three categories: reexperiencing (e.g., recurring nightmares about the traumatic event); avoidance (e.g., avoiding conversations about the traumatic event); and arousal (e.g., difficulty sleeping). Symptoms must persist for at least one month and must result in clinically significant distress or impairment in functioning.[12]

Figure 2 shows the prevalence of PTSD among OEF/OIF veterans receiving VA health of Public Health care in FY2002-FY2010.[13] This percentage is subject to important data limitations discussed in **Appendix A.**

PTSD Treatment in the VA Health Care System

Department policy requires that veterans new to VA health care receive a PTSD screening, which is repeated every year for the first five years and every five years thereafter, unless there is a clinical need to screen earlier. Department policy also requires that new patients requesting or referred for mental health services receive an initial assessment within 24 hours and a full evaluation appointment within 14 days; follow-up appointments for established patients must occur within 30 days.[14] Congressional testimony has raised questions about the extent to which these policies are implemented in practice.[15]

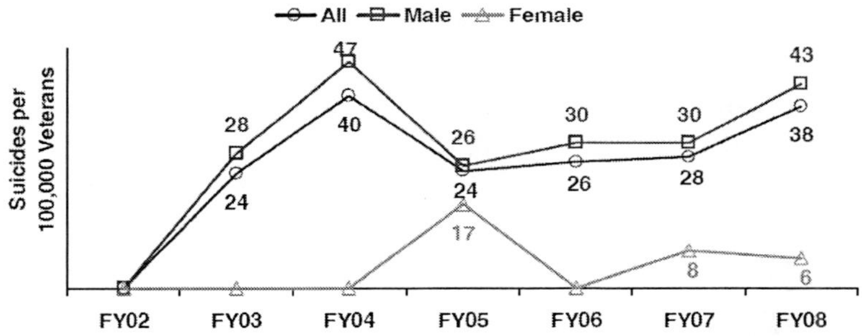

Source: CRS analysis of data provided by the VA on March 8, 2011, pursuant to a CRS inquiry.

Note: Rates are presented per 100,000 OEF/OIF veterans enrolled in VA health care; for example, in FY2008, the rate of suicides was 38 per 100,000 OEF/OIF veterans (male and female) enrolled in VA health care.

Figure 1. Annual Suicides per 100,000 OEF/OIFVeterans Using VA Health Care, FY2002-FY2008.

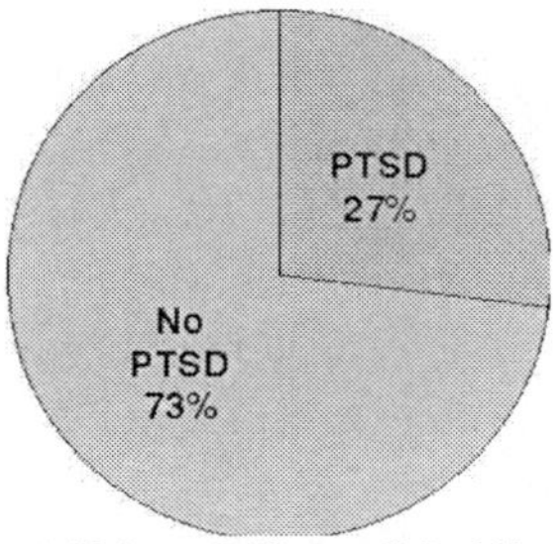

Source: U.S. Department of Veterans Affairs, Office of Public Health and Environmental Hazards, *Analysis of VA Health Care Utilization Among Operation Enduring Freedom (OEF) and Operation Iraqi Freedom (OIF) Veterans, Cumulative from 1st Quarter FY2002 Through 4th Quarter FY2010*, December 2010.

Figure 2. Prevalence of PTSD Among OEF/OIF Veterans Using VA Health Care, FY2002-FY2010.

PTSD treatment provided by the VA includes both medication and cognitive-behavioral therapy (a category of talk therapy).[16] Every VA Medical Center has specialists in PTSD treatment. Some facilities offer specialized PTSD treatment programs of varying intensity and duration, including (among others) PTSD day hospitals (four to eight hours per day, several days per week); evaluation and brief treatment PTSD units (14-28 days); specialized inpatient PTSD units (28-90 days); and PTSD residential rehabilitation programs (28-90 days living in a supportive environment while receiving treatment). Veterans may also receive PTSD treatment at VA community-based outpatient clinics (CBOCs)[17] or at Vet Centers[18] (which are subject to different policies than VA health care facilities).[19] Several reports that have evaluated the VA's PTSD screening and treatment efforts, and offered recommendations, are listed in **Appendix B**.

SUBSTANCE USE DISORDERS

Substance use disorders include dependence on and abuse of drugs, alcohol, or other substances (e.g., nicotine). A diagnosis of dependence requires at least three symptoms (e.g., tolerance or withdrawal); substance use that does not meet criteria for dependence, but leads to clinically significant distress or impairment, is called abuse.[20] Each diagnosis is specific to the substance, so an individual may have multiple diagnoses of abuse or dependence—one for each substance (e.g., marijuana dependence and cocaine abuse).

Figure 3 shows the prevalence of drug dependence and abuse among OEF/OIF veterans using VA health care during FY2002-FY2010.[21] Alcohol dependence (7%) is more common than either drug dependence or abuse; the prevalence of alcohol abuse was not provided. These percentages are subject toimportant data limitations discussed in **Appendix A**.

Substance Use Disorder Treatment in the VA Health Care System

Given the comparatively low rates of drug abuse and dependence (relative to PTSD or alcohol dependence), VA policy does not require routine drug use screening. Department policy does require an annual alcohol screening, which is waived for veterans who drank no alcohol in the prior year.[22]

The VA offers medication and psychosocial interventions for substance use disorders, as well as acute detoxification care when necessary. Medication may be used to reduce cravings or to substitute for the drug of abuse (e.g., methadone for heroin users). Psychosocial interventions include (among others) brief counseling to enhance motivation to change; intensive outpatient treatment (i.e., at least nine hours of treatment per week); residential care (i.e., living in a supportive environment while receiving treatment); long-term relapse prevention; and referral to outside programs such as Alcoholics Anonymous.[23]

Several reports that have evaluated the department's alcohol screening and substance use disorder treatment efforts, and offered recommendations, are listed in **Appendix B**.

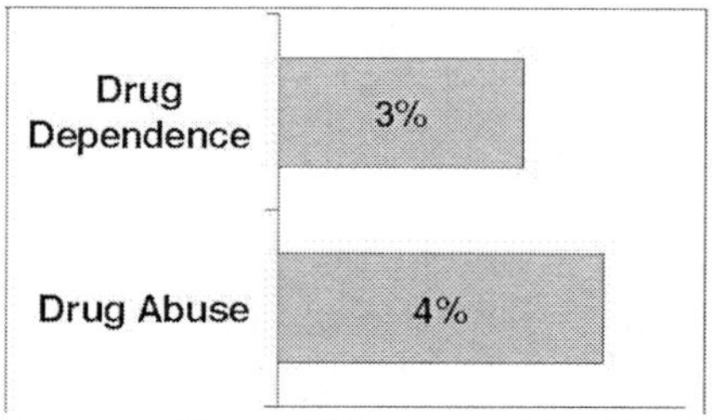

Source: U.S. Department of Veterans Affairs, Office of Public Health and Environmental Hazards, *Analysis of VA Health Care Utilization Among Operation Enduring Freedom (OEF) and Operation Iraqi Freedom (OIF) Veterans, Cumulative from 1st Quarter FY2002 Through 4th Quarter FY2010*, December 2010.

Figure 3. Prevalence of Drug Abuse and Dependence Among OEF/OIF Veterans Using VA Health Care, FY2002-FY2010.

APPENDIX A. DATA LIMITATIONS

In order to understand the limitations of the data presented in this report, it is helpful to understand their sources. As noted previously, the VA identifies veteran suicides by matching suicides from the National Death Index with the roster of veterans in VA administrative data. The VA identifies PTSD and substance use disorders by searching VA administrative data for diagnosis codes associated with specific conditions (e.g., 309.81 for PTSD). These codes are entered into veterans' electronic medical records by clinicians, in the normal course of evaluation and treatment.

The data provided by the VA should be interpreted in light of at least four limitations, each of which is discussed below.

First, suicides may be understated, because cause of death might not always be accurately identified in the National Death Index, particularly where intent is involved. For example, it may not be known whether a car crash or drug overdose is intentional, which may be the determining factor in identifying suicide.

Second, some conditions may be overstated, because veterans with diagnosis codes for a condition might not have the condition, as a result of provisional diagnoses or noncurrent diagnoses. A provisional diagnosis code may be entered into a veteran's electronic medical record when further evaluation is required to confirm the diagnosis. A diagnosis may be noncurrent when a veteran who had a condition in the past no longer has it. In either case, the code remains in the veteran's electronic medical record.

Third, some conditions may be understated, because veterans who have a condition might not be diagnosed (and therefore might not have the diagnosis code in their records), if they choose not to disclose their symptoms. Veterans might not want to disclose information that would lead to a diagnosis of mental illness. Veterans have reported not wanting to disclose trauma for fear that that they will not be believed, that others will think less of them, that they will be institutionalized or stigmatized, or that their careers will be jeopardized, among other reasons.[24] Also, veterans using VA health care services may receive additional services outside the VA, without the knowledge of the department.

Fourth, the numbers provided by the VA should not be extrapolated to all OEF/OIF veterans, or to the broader veteran population, because OEF/OIF veterans using VA health care are not representative of all OEF/OIF veterans or the broader veteran population. Veterans who use VA health care may differ from those who do not, in ways that are not known. Potential differences include (among other characteristics) disability status, employment status, and distance from a VA medical facility.

APPENDIX B. SELECTED EVALUATIONS OF VA SERVICES

Table B-1 lists selected reports published since 2008 that evaluate VA's efforts to address suicide, PTSD, and substance use disorders. In some cases, the focus of the evaluation was broader than the specific topics addressed in this report (e.g., mental health services generally).

Table B-1. Selected Evaluations of VA Mental Health Services Since 2008

Report Full Citation and Link	Suicide	PTSD	Substance Use
Department of Veterans Affairs, Office of Inspector General, *Healthcare Inspection: Post Traumatic Stress Disorder Counseling Services at Vet Centers*, Report No. 10-00628-170, May 17, 2011, http://www.va.gov/oig/54/reports/ VAOIG-10-00628-170.pdf		√	
Department of Veterans Affairs, Office of Inspector General, Combined Assessment Program Summary Report Re-Evaluation of Suicide Prevention Safety Plan Practices in Veterans Health Administration Facilities, Report Number 11-01380-128, March 22, 2011, http://www.va.gov/oig/CAP/ VAOIG-11-01380-128. pdf	√		
Department of Veterans Affairs, Office of Inspector General, *Healthcare Inspection: Progress in Implementing the Veterans Health Administration's Uniform Mental Health Services Handbook*, Report No. 08-02917-145, May 4, 2010, http:// www.va.gov/oig/54/reports/VAOIG-08-02917-145.pdf	√	√	√
U.S. Government Accountability Office, *VA Faces Challenges in Providing Substance Use Disorder Services and Is Taking Steps to Improve These Services for Veterans*, GAO-10-294R, March 10, 2010, http://www.gao.gov/new. items/d10294r.pdf			√
Department of Veterans Affairs, Office of Inspector General, Healthcare Inspection: Evaluation of Suicide Prevention Program Implementation in Veterans Health Administration Facilities January–June, 2009, Report Number 09-00326-223, September 22, 2009, http://www.va.gov/oig/54/reports/ VAOIG-09-00326-223.pdf	√		
Department of Veterans Affairs, Office of Inspector General, *Healthcare Inspection: Review of Veterans Health Administration Residential Mental Health Care Facilities*, Report No. 08-00038-152, June 25, 2009, http://www.va.gov/oig/54/ reports/VAOIG-08-00038-152.pdf		√	√
Blue Ribbon Work Group on Suicide Prevention in the Veteran Population, *Report to James B. Peake, MD, Secretary of Veterans Affairs*, June 30, 2008, http://www.mental health.va. gov/suicide_prevention/Blue_Ribbon_ Report-FINAL_June-30-08.pdf	√		

Source: CRS search for evaluations of VA services related to suicide, PTSD, and substance use, since 2008.

End Notes

[1] *Veterans for Common Sense v. Shinseki*, No. 08-16728 6 (U.S. 9th Circuit Court of Appeals 2011).
[2] The suit also addressed VA's handling of disability benefits claims and medical services.
[3] Operation Enduring Freedom (OEF) began on October 7, 2001, and continues today. Operation Iraqi Freedom (OIF) began on March 20, 2003. On September 1, 2010, OIF was redesignated Operation New Dawn, which continues today. The beginning dates of these operations are not defined in statute; the dates presented are commonly accepted. In this report, the abbreviation OEF/OIF refers to Operation Enduring Freedom and Operation Iraqi Freedom, including Operation New Dawn.
[4] Summary of CRS Report R41343, *Veterans Medical Care: FY2011 Appropriations*, by Sidath Viranga Panangala.
[5] Under the National Defense Authorization Act for Fiscal Year 2008 (P.L. 110-181), OEF/OIF veterans discharged or released from active service on or after January 28, 2003, are eligible to enroll in the VA health care system for five years from the date of discharge or release. They continue to be enrolled after the five-year eligibility period ends.
[6] Department of Veterans Affairs, Office of Public Health and Environmental Hazards, *Analysis of VA Health Care Utilization among Operation Enduring Freedom (OEF) and Operation Iraqi Freedom (OIF) Veterans, Cumulative from 1st Quarter FY2002 through 4th Quarter FY2010*, December 2010.
[7] Prevalence is the percentage of a specified population experiencing a condition within a given timeframe.
[8] Using the Federal Health and Bi-directional Health Information Exchange (FHIE/BHIE), VA and DOD share most essential health information that is available in electronic form.
[9] For more information, see Centers for Disease Control and Prevention, National Center for Health Statistics, *About the National Death Index*, http://www.cdc.gov/nchs/data_access/ ndi/about_ndi.htm.
[10] The suicide rate is the ratio of the number of OEF/OIF veterans enrolled in VA health care who are identified as suicides in the NDI during the year to the total number of OEF/OIF veterans enrolled in VA health care (whether in active treatment or not). The result is then multiplied by 100,000 to create a rate per 100,000 OEF/OIF veterans.
[11] Department of Veterans Affairs, *Suicide Prevention*, http://www.mentalhealth.va.gov/suicide_ prevention/.
[12] CRS summary of American Psychiatric Association, *Diagnostic and Statistical Manual of Mental Disorders, Fourth Edition, Text Revision* (Washington, DC: American Psychiatric Association, 2000), pp. 467-468.
[13] Prevalence is the ratio of the number of OEF/OIF veterans with a diagnosis code indicating PTSD in FY2002-FY2010 to the number of OEF/OIF veterans enrolled in VA health care in FY2002-FY2010.
[14] Department of Veterans Affairs, Veterans Health Administration, *Programs for Veterans with Post-Traumatic Stress Disorder (PTSD)*, VHA Handbook 1160.03, March 12, 2010.
[15] U.S. Congress, Senate Committee on Veterans' Affairs, *VA Mental Health Care: Closing the Gaps*, 112th Cong., 1st sess., July 14, 2011.
[16] Jessica Hamblen, *Treatment of PTSD*, Department of Veterans Affairs, National Center for PTSD, 2010.
[17] For more information on CBOCs see CRS Report R41044, *Veterans Health Administration: Community-Based Outpatient Clinics*, by Sidath Viranga Panangala.
[18] Readjustment Counseling Centers (Vet Centers) provide veterans and their families with services such as screening and counseling for PTSD or substance use disorders, employment/educational counseling, bereavement counseling, military sexual trauma counseling, and marital and family counseling.
[19] Department of Veterans Affairs, National Center for PTSD, *PTSD Treatment Programs in the U.S. Department of Veterans Affairs*, http://www.ptsd.va.gov/public/pages/va-ptsd-treatment-programs.asp.
[20] CRS summary of American Psychiatric Association, *Diagnostic and Statistical Manual of Mental Disorders, Fourth Edition, Text Revision* (Washington, DC: American Psychiatric Association, 2000), pp. 191-199.
[21] Prevalence is the ratio of the number of OEF/OIF veterans with a diagnosis code indicating abuse/dependence inFY2002-FY2010 to the number of OEF/OIF veterans enrolled in VA health care in FY2002-FY2010.
[22] Department of Veterans Affairs and Department of Defense, *VA/DOD Clinical Practice Guideline for the Management of Substance Use Disorders*, August 2009.
[23] Department of Veterans Affairs, *Summary of VA Treatment Programs for Substance Use Problems*, May 20, 2010, http://www.mentalhealth.va.gov/res-vatreatmentprograms.asp.
[24] Matthew D Jeffreys, Ruth Q Leibowitz, Erin Finley, et al., "Trauma Disclosure to Health Care Professionals by Veterans: Clinical Implications," *Military Medicine*, vol. 175, no. 10 (October 2010), pp. 719-724.

In: Veteran Injuries, Disorders and Medical Care Service
Editors: Jessica Michaels and Jesse E. Levine
ISBN: 978-1-62081-302-7

Chapter 4

TRAUMATIC BRAIN INJURY AMONG VETERANS*

Erin Bagalman

SUMMARY

Traumatic Brain Injury (TBI) has been defined as "an alteration in brain function, or other evidence of brain pathology, caused by an external force." In the general population, TBI results mainly from falls, motor vehicle/traffic accidents, assaults, and other instances in which the head is struck by or strikes against an object. In military servicemembers, TBI may also result from improvised explosive devices, mortars, grenades, bullets, or mines.

Traumatic brain injury has become known as a "signature wound" of Operation Enduring Freedom (OEF) and Operation Iraqi Freedom (OIF), because the incidence of TBI is higher in these conflicts than it has been in previous conflicts. As of FY2010, 1.25 million OEF/OIF veterans have left active duty and became eligible for Department of Veterans Affairs (VA) health care; half of them have obtained VA health care; and 45,606 have been diagnosed with TBI-related conditions at VA medical facilities. The total number of OEF/OIF veterans with TBI is not known, in part because some OEF/OIF veterans have not accessed VA health care services.

The VA has engaged in outreach efforts to OEF/OIF veterans via mail, telephone, and television advertisements. In order to make contact with servicemembers before separation and conversion to veteran status, the VA participates in some Department of Defense (DOD) activities. Some OEF/OIF veterans may choose not to enroll in VA health care, because they have health coverage from other sources or because they do not perceive a need for health care. Others may experience barriers to accessing VA care.

Servicemembers who sustain mild TBI (also known as "concussion"), which accounts for the majority of injuries, may walk away from the event, seemingly unharmed; thus mild TBI may go unnoticed and untreated. Accordingly, VA policy requires that all OEF/OIF veterans receiving medical care in the VA health care system must be screened for possible TBI, and that those who screen positive must be offered further evaluation and specialized treatment.

* This is an edited, reformatted and augmented version of the Congressional Research Service Publication, CRS Report for Congress R40941, dated May 5, 2011 .

The VA and the DOD have jointly developed evidence-based clinical practice guidelines for treatment of mild TBI.

Servicemembers who sustain moderate to severe TBI (i.e., recognizable injuries) require immediate treatment, which begins at the site of the event and continues at a military treatment facility. Once stabilized, servicemembers may remain at a military treatment facility or be transferred to the VA Polytrauma System of Care. Transfers from DOD to VA facilities require coordination between the two systems, and several programs have been developed to facilitate coordination of care.

The VA's FY2010 budget for "TBI and Other Neurotrauma" research was $22 million (rounded). Before applying a 0.2% rescission for most non-defense items, the full-year continuing resolution for FY2011 maintained VA's research funding at the FY2010 level. The large number of studies conducted by the VA and the DOD, as well as the Department of Health and Human Services (HHS), raises questions for some about potential duplication of effort, gaps in the research, dissemination of research findings, and translation of research into practice.

INTRODUCTION

Traumatic brain injury (TBI) has become known as a "signature wound" of Operation Enduring Freedom (OEF) and Operation Iraqi Freedom (OIF),[1] because the incidence of TBI is higher in these conflicts than it has been in previous conflicts. This report discusses TBI among veterans receiving care in Department of Veterans Affairs (VA) medical facilities, with particular attention to OEF/OIF veterans.

The VA health care system does not function in a vacuum. Individuals may sustain injuries during military service, receive early stages of treatment from the Department of Defense (DOD), and transfer to the VA for later stages of treatment. In this report, agencies other than the VA are addressed only to the extent that they work in coordination with the VA.

The remainder of this report is organized in three parts. The first part provides an overview of TBI, as background for the rest of the report. The second part focuses on TBI among veterans receiving VA health care services,[2] with sections addressing access to care, identification of TBI, treatment of TBI, and TBI research. The third part discusses potential issues for the 112th Congress, in the context of past congressional action related to TBI among veterans.

Several numbers are presented in this report, quantifying TBI among different populations (i.e., civilians, servicemembers, or veterans), measured over different periods (i.e., a single year or multiple years), by different organizations (i.e., the Centers for Disease Control and Prevention, DOD, or VA). Each number is independent of the others; they do not sum to a total.

TRAUMATIC BRAIN INJURY (TBI) OVERVIEW

To provide some context for the discussion of TBI among veterans, this part of the report discusses TBI in general terms, including the definition, causes, and prevalence of TBI; various ways in which traumatic brain injuries can be classified; the signs and symptoms of TBI; and associated comorbid conditions (including both mental and physical health).

Definition, Causes, and Prevalence

In 2011, the Brain Injury Association of America adopted a definition of TBI as "an alteration in brain function, or other evidence of brain pathology, caused by an external force."[3] In the general population, TBI results mainly from falls, motor vehicle/traffic accidents, assaults, and other instances in which the head is struck by or strikes against an object.[4] In the United States each year, an estimated 1.7 million people sustain TBI:

- 1.365 million are treated and released from an emergency department,
- 275,000 are hospitalized, and
- 52,000 die as a result of their injuries.

In military servicemembers, TBI may result from the events listed above, or from improvised explosive devices, mortars, grenades, bullets, or mines.[5] The DOD reports that in 2010, a total of 30,703 servicemembers sustained TBI.[6]

Classification

Traumatic brain injury is not a specific diagnosis; the term encompasses a range of conditions. A TBI may be classified as focal or diffuse; open or closed; and mild, moderate, or severe. If the injury is localized to a small area of the brain, it is a focal injury; an injury occurring over a large area is diffuse. If the head hits, or is hit by, an object that penetrates the skull and the brain's protective coverings, the injury is open (also called penetrating); otherwise, the injury is closed and can be further classified as mild, moderate, or severe.[7]

Many methods have been used to classify TBI as mild, moderate, or severe; three commonly used methods are based on loss of consciousness, post-traumatic amnesia (i.e., loss of memory), or the Glasgow Coma Scale.[8] The Glasgow Coma Scale assigns points in three areas: eye opening, verbal response, and motor response. The sum of points in the three areas ranges from 3 to 15, with lower scores indicating greater severity of TBI.[9] **Table 1** summarizes the criteria for mild, moderate, and severe TBI.

Table 1. Classification of TBI as Mild, Moderate, or Severe

	Mild	Moderate	Severe
Loss of consciousness	< 30 minutes	30 minutes-24 hours	> 24 hours
Post-traumatic amnesia	< 1 day	1-7 days	> 7 days
Glasgow Coma Scale score	13-15 points	9-12 points	3-8 points (coma)

Source: CRS summary of classification described by Michael S. Jaffee, Kathy M. Helmick, and Philip D. Girard, et al., "Acute clinical care and care coordination within Department of Defense," *Journal of Rehabilitation Research & Development*, vol. 46, no. 6 (2009), pp. 655-666.

Signs and Symptoms

Mild TBI (concussion) may manifest as a range of physical, psychological, and cognitive problems. Common physical signs and symptoms of mild TBI include headaches, fatigue, lethargy, dizziness, and lightheadedness. Individuals with mild TBI may experience blurred vision, eye fatigue, ringing in the ears, or a bad taste in the mouth. Psychological symptoms may appear as behavioral or mood changes. Cognitive difficulties may include confusion and problems with memory, attention, concentration, or thinking. Individuals with mild TBI may also sleep more or less than usual.[10]

Individuals with moderate to severe TBI may experience any of the signs and symptoms listed above, as well as repeated nausea or vomiting, a persistent or worsening headache, seizures or convulsions, numbness or weakness in their feet or hands, and loss of coordination. They may experience increased confusion, restlessness, or agitation. Their pupils might be dilated and their speech might be slurred. They may be unable to awaken from sleep.[11]

Comorbid Conditions

Traumatic brain injury is associated with comorbid conditions that include both mental and physical illnesses. Mental disorders associated with TBI include anxiety disorders and depressive disorders; estimates of how often such conditions co-occur with TBI vary.[12] While some studies have found a link between TBI and increased alcohol or drug use, a report by the Institute of Medicine (IOM) found just the opposite: limited/suggestive evidence of an association between TBI and decreased alcohol and drug use within one to three years of the injury.[13]

Individuals with TBI are at increased risk of developing epilepsy and neurodegenerative diseases such as Alzheimer's disease, Lewy body dementia, or Parkinson's disease. Repetitive blows to the head can result in chronic traumatic encephalopathy (CTE); CTE may begin with loss of concentration, attention, or memory, and may eventually progress to problems with coordination, gait, slurred speech, and tremors. Post-traumatic hypopituitarism (PTH) is a neuroendocrine disorder associated with TBI; chronic PTH leads to other neuroendocrine conditions, including hypothyroidism and deficiencies in growth hormone and gonadotropin. Individuals with TBI may also develop sleep disturbances, obstructive sleep apnea, incontinence, sexual dysfunction, metabolic dysfunction, or musculoskeletal dysfunction.[14]

The next part of the report addresses TBI in the veteran population, including sections on access to care, identification of TBI, treatment of TBI, and TBI research.

TBI AMONG VETERANS

As stated before, traumatic brain injury has become known as a "signature wound" of OEF/OIF, because servicemembers in these operations have experienced TBI in larger numbers than those serving in past conflicts. Three factors contribute to the increase in TBI. First, the number of blast injuries caused by improvised explosive devices (IED), rocket-propelled grenades, and land mines has increased; it has been reported that the primary mechanism of injury in OIF is a blast injury.[15] Second, injuries that would have been fatal in the past may not be fatal now, thanks to advances in protective equipment, combat medicine, and air evacuation.[16] Third, health care professionals are more alert to the possibility of TBI and may therefore be more likely to diagnose TBI accurately.[17]

The total number of veterans who have experienced TBI is not known, in part because TBI is difficult to identify,[18] and in part because some veterans have not accessed VA health care services.[19] Among OEF/OIF veterans who have accessed VA health care services, the VA has indicated that 45,606 have been diagnosed with TBI-related conditions at VA medical facilities as of FY2010.[20] The number in each state is shown in **Appendix A**.

This part of the report focuses on TBI among veterans receiving care provided by VA medical facilities. The four sections address access to care, identification of TBI, treatment of TBI, and TBI research. Because individuals may sustain injuries during military service (as noted previously), the DOD may have a role in each of these areas; however, as noted previously, the focus of this report is on the VA, and other agencies are addressed only to the extent that they work in coordination with the VA.

Access to Care

This section summarizes enrollment in VA health care and briefly describes VA outreach efforts to increase enrollment.

Veterans generally must enroll in the VA health care system to receive medical care, as described in the text box below.

The VA has engaged in outreach efforts to OEF/OIF veterans via mail,[21] telephone,[22] and television advertisements.[23] In order to make contact with servicemembers before separation and conversion to veteran status, the VA participates in some DOD activities. VA reaches out to OEF/OIF veterans to inform them of their benefits by

- participating in Reserve component out-processing at DOD demobilization sites;
- attending the DOD's Yellow Ribbon Program (YRP) events;[24]
- partnering with the National Guard in training transition assistance advisors;
- contacting OEF/OIF veterans through the Combat Veterans Call Center;

- supporting the DOD health assessment and linking veterans with appointments;
- hosting Individual Ready Reserve musters; and
- using social media and other internet-based outreach.[25]

From FY2002 through FY2010, 1.25 million OEF/OIF veterans (including members of the Reserve and National Guard) left active duty and became eligible for VA health care; by the end of FY2010, half of them had obtained VA health care.[26] Some veterans may choose not to enroll in VA health care because they have health coverage from other sources (e.g., private insurance or TRICARE[27]) or because they do not perceive a need for health care. Others may experience barriers to accessing VA care; potential barriers to access are discussed under "Potential Issues for the 112th Congress" later in this report.

Identification of TBI

This section describes the two-step process the VA uses to identify TBI: screening for TBI and confirming a diagnosis of TBI.

As noted previously, the initial injury may occur during military service; thus the DOD may be responsible for identification of TBI. Moderate to severe TBI, in particular, is likely to be recognized immediately at the time of the initial injury; however, mild TBI may go unnoticed if an individual walks away seemingly unharmed. Despite repeated assessments by the DOD, a veteran may enter the VA health care system with an undiagnosed TBI. In order to identify cases of TBI that might otherwise go untreated, VA policy requires that all OEF/OIF veterans receiving medical care in the VA health care system must be screened for possible TBI, and that those who screen positive must be offered further evaluation and specialized treatment.[28]

The VA developed a screening instrument and a protocol for further evaluation of individuals who screen positive. The screening instrument was adapted from one already used by the DOD and was incorporated into a national clinical reminder in the computerized patient record system.[29] When a provider opens a veteran's computerized record, the clinical reminder alerts the provider that action is required. The clinical reminder then prompts the provider to ask the veteran a series of questions in order to complete the TBI screening instrument.

If a veteran screens negative for possible TBI, the clinical reminder is resolved and no further action is required. If a veteran screens positive for possible TBI, the clinical reminder generates an electronic consult for a follow-up evaluation. The protocol for completing the additional evaluation includes a 22-item neurobehavioral symptom inventory.

The diagnosis of TBI is complicated by symptoms that overlap with posttraumatic stress disorder (PTSD),[30] such as difficulty concentrating, irritability or outbursts of anger, and memory loss.[31] Because of the complexity of diagnosing TBI and differentiating symptoms of other disorders,[32] specialized training is required to administer the evaluation.[33]

If the follow-up evaluation finds that the veteran does not have TBI, the consult is completed and results are reported to the referring clinician. If the follow-up evaluation finds that the veteran has TBI, the veteran is referred for specialized treatment, as described in the next section.

Veterans Health Administration: Eligibility, Enrollment, and Services

The Department of Veterans Affairs (VA) provides services and benefits to eligible veterans through three major operating units: the Veterans Health Administration (VHA), the Veterans Benefits Administration (VBA), and the National Cemetery Administration (NCA). The VHA operates the nation's largest integrated direct health care delivery system. As of FY2010, the VHA health care system includes 152 hospitals (medical centers), 133 nursing homes, 791 community-based outpatient clinics (CBOCs), and 6 independent outpatient clinics. (The VHA also operates 300 Readjustment Counseling Centers, or Vet Centers, which provide psychosocial services, but not medical care; Vet Centers have their own eligibility criteria.)

Under the Veterans' Health Care Eligibility Reform Act of 1996 (P.L. 104-262), eligibility for VHA health care is based primarily on veteran status, which is established by a period of active-duty status and an honorable discharge or release from active military service. (A veteran with a discharge other than honorable may still retain eligibility for VA health care benefits for disabilities incurred or aggravated during service in the military.) As a requirement to obtain care through the VA, veterans are required to enroll in the VA health care system. Once enrolled, veterans are categorized into eight priority groups. Veterans with service-connected disabilities or with incomes below a means test are designated "high priority" and are enrolled in Priority Groups 1-6. (The term "service-connected" means, with respect to disability, that such disability was incurred or aggravated in the line of duty in the active military, naval, or air service.) The remaining veterans (primarily those without service-connected medical conditions and with incomes and net worth above the means test) are enrolled in Priority Group 7 or 8.

Under the National Defense Authorization Act for Fiscal Year 2008 (P.L. 110-181), veterans who served in a theater of combat operations after November 11, 1998, are offered a five-year post-discharge period of enhanced enrollment for VHA health care. Veterans who enroll during this period are provided care regardless of service-connected disability status. Veterans who enroll in the VHA system under this extended enrollment authority continue to be enrolled even after the five-year eligibility period ends.

In FY2010 approximately 8.4 million veterans were enrolled in the VHA health care system; this represents 36.4% of the 23.1 million veterans living in the United States. Thus the majority of veterans (63.6%) are not enrolled in the VHA health care system.

All enrolled veterans are offered a standard medical benefits package, which includes a full range of inpatient, outpatient, and preventive medical services. Among these services are medical, surgical, and mental health care, including substance abuse treatment; prescription drugs, including over-the-counter drugs, available under the VA national formulary system; home health services and institutional respite care; noninstitutional adult day health care and noninstitutional respite care; and periodic medical exams.

Source: Summarized from CRS Report R41343, *Veterans Medical Care: FY2011 Appropriations*.
Note: Some of the numbers have been updated since publication of the source report.

As of September 2010, a total of 420,374 OEF/OIF veterans had been screened for TBI. Of those who were screened, 102,569 either reported a prior diagnosis of TBI or screened positive for possible TBI. A follow-up evaluation (which was not required for those who reported a prior diagnosis of TBI) was completed for 57,995 of those who screened positive for possible TBI, and a TBI diagnosis was confirmed in 18,280 of them.[34] Note that the 18,280 represents only those OEF/OIF veterans with a TBI diagnosis confirmed by the VA's follow-up evaluation. It does not include OEF/OIF veterans who reported a prior diagnosis of TBI at the screening, nor does it include OEF/OIF veterans who do not receive VA health care.

The VA's identification process is illustrated in **Appendix B** (which also illustrates the treatment process that follows).

Treatment of TBI

This section describes treatment of veterans with TBI in the VA health care system, focusing on treatment of veterans with moderate to severe TBI. The first subsection describes the VA Polytrauma System of Care. The second subsection describes several programs aimed at coordinating VA and DOD treatment.

As mentioned previously, the early stages of treatment may occur within the military health care system, if the initial injury occurs during military service; however, this report focuses on treatment within the VA health care system. Regardless of where treatment is provided, the type of treatment needed depends on the severity of the injury.

Servicemembers who sustain mild TBI (which accounts for the majority of injuries[35]) may walk away from the event, seemingly unharmed; thus mild TBI may go unnoticed and untreated. Most cases of mild TBI resolve without medical attention. Education about mild TBI can effectively "normalize symptoms and provide expectation of rapid recovery."[36] The VA and the DOD have jointly developed evidence-based clinical practice guidelines for treatment of mild TBI.[37]

Servicemembers who sustain moderate to severe TBI (i.e., recognizable injuries) require immediate treatment, which begins at the site of the event and continues at a military treatment facility. Once stabilized, servicemembers may remain at a military treatment facility or be sent to VA medical facilities for continuing treatment, rehabilitation, and transitional care. When servicemembers transfer from DOD to VA facilities (regardless of whether they change to veteran status), coordination between the two systems is necessary.

VA Polytrauma System of Care

Veterans with moderate to severe TBI (alone or in combination with other conditions) may receive care through the VA Polytrauma System of Care (PSC).[38] The PSC is designed to function within the existing VA health care system, which is organized into geographic regions called Veterans Integrated Service Networks (VISN). Like the larger VISN structure, the PSC is geographically dispersed, thereby making the specialized treatment more accessible to veterans, regardless of where they live. The PSC operates as a "hub and spoke" model with four components, each of which is described below.

Component I of the PSC comprises four regional Polytrauma Rehabilitation Centers, which serve as regional referral centers, the "hubs" of the PSC. Polytrauma Rehabilitation

Centers provide direct care and consultation, as well as research and education related to polytrauma and TBI. Each Polytrauma Rehabilitation Center has a minimum of 12 dedicated comprehensive rehabilitation beds and 10 dedicated transitional rehabilitation beds. Required staff include a rehabilitation physician, registered nurses, social workers, speech-language pathologists, physical therapists, occupational therapists, recreation therapists, a neuropsychologist, a counseling psychologist, and a family therapist, among others. Construction of a fifth regional Polytrauma Rehabilitation Center is underway.

Component II of the PSC extends the "spokes" to 22 Polytrauma Network Sites: one in each VISN (including one at each of the Polytrauma Rehabilitation Centers) plus one in Puerto Rico. In consultation with the Polytrauma Rehabilitation Centers, Polytrauma Network Sites provide specialized, post-acute rehabilitation services in a setting appropriate to the needs of veterans, servicemembers, and families. Each Polytrauma Network Site has a dedicated interdisciplinary team with specialized training, to provide case management and identify resources both within and outside the VA. **Figure 1** shows the location of each Polytrauma Network Site, including the Polytrauma Rehabilitation Centers.

Component III of the PSC extends care to 82 VA medical facilities that do not have Polytrauma Rehabilitation Centers or Polytrauma Network Sites, by establishing Polytrauma Support Clinic Teams. These local teams of providers have rehabilitation expertise and deliver follow-up services in consultation with regional and network specialists. They provide direct care, consultation, and telerehabilitation, as needed.

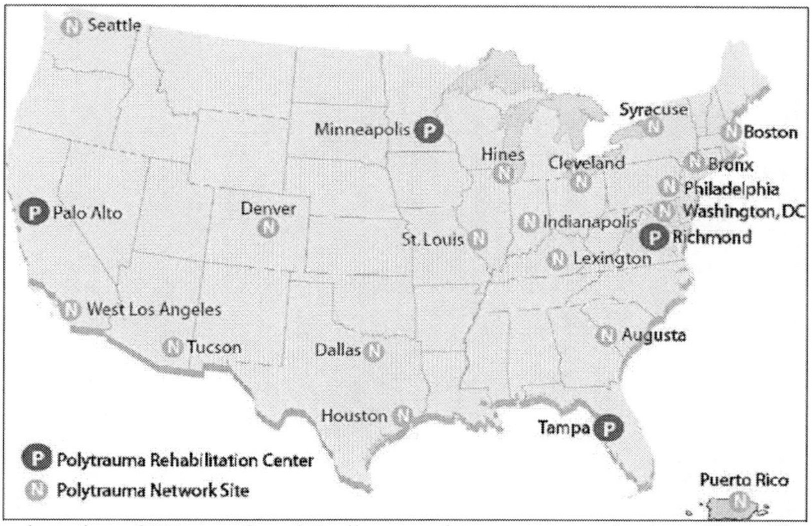

Source: CRS adaptation of VA map from http://www.polytrauma.va.gov/system-of-care/care-facilities.
Note: A fifth Polytrauma Rehabilitation Center is currently under construction in San Antonio, TX.

Figure 1.VA Polytrauma System of Care
Location of Polytrauma Rehabilitation Centers and Polytrauma Network Sites.

Component IV of the PSC addresses the needs of veterans at 48 VA medical facilities that lack the necessary services to provide specialized care. Such facilities must designate a Polytrauma Point of Contact who is responsible for coordinating the treatment of veterans at their facility. The role of the Polytrauma Point of Contact is to ensure that veterans are referred to a facility capable of providing the services they require.

The treatment process within the VA's PSC (excluding any treatment provided by the DOD) is illustrated in **Appendix B**, which also illustrates the identification process described earlier.

Coordination of VA and DOD Treatment

As noted elsewhere in this report, injured servicemembers may transfer directly from military treatment facilities to VA medical facilities (and may later convert to veteran status), or veterans may access VA medical facilities after having received treatment in military facilities. Such situations require coordination between the two agencies in caring for servicemembers or veterans with TBI. Three VA and joint VA/DOD programs seek to address the transition from DOD to VA health care facilities: OEF/OIF Care Management, the VA Liaison Program, and the Federal Recovery Coordinator Program.[39]

Every VA Medical Center has an OEF/OIF Care Management Team, consisting of case managers and transition patient advocates, to help coordinate care and navigate the VA system. Case managers are either nurses or social workers. Transition patient advocates serve as personal advocates for patients moving throughout the VA health care system. This service is available to all OEF/OIF veterans without referral.

The VA Liaison Program places VA employees at military treatment facilities, where they provide onsite consultation about VA resources. Liaisons coordinate referrals with the OEF/OIF Care Management teams at local VA facilities; they maintain involvement until health care is arranged and transfer is complete. **Figure 2** shows the locations of military treatment facilities with VA liaisons and the number of liaisons at each facility.

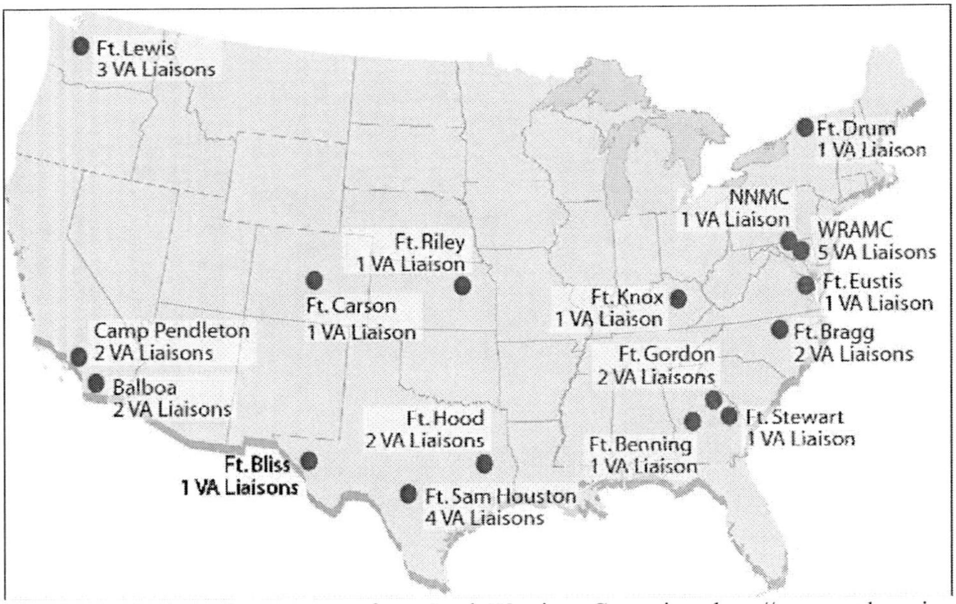

Source: CRS adaptation of DOD map from Real Warriors Campaign, http://www.realwarriors.net/guardreserve/ reintegration/VAbenefits.php

Notes: NNMC = National Naval Medical Center; WRAMC = Walter Reed Army Medical Center.

Figure 2. Locations of VA Liaisons Assigned to Military Treatment Facilities.

The Federal Recovery Coordination Program (FRCP) was established via a memorandum of understanding between the VA and the DOD, signed on October 30, 2007.[40] Veterans or servicemembers with TBI (one of several qualifying conditions) can self-refer to the FRCP or be referred by clinicians, family members, veterans service organizations, or others. Each veteran (or servicemember) enrolled in the FRCP is assigned a Federal Recovery Coordinator (FRC), who coordinates services provided by the DOD, the VA, and other public and private entities; the FRC does not provide direct services.

TBI Research

The VA's FY2010 budget for "TBI and Other Neurotrauma" research was $22 million (rounded).[41] Before applying a 0.2% rescission for most non-defense items, the full-year continuing resolution for FY2011 maintained VA's research funding at the FY2010 level.[42]

The VA Office of Research and Development has solicited research proposals on a range of topics related to TBI, including (but not limited to)

- identifying the origins, disease pathways, and genetics of TBI;
- operationalizing the definition of mild TBI;
- developing and evaluating instruments to measure TBI;
- assessing the service needs of veterans with TBI and barriers to treatment; and
- identifying and evaluating treatments for TBI.[43]

Research on TBI and related conditions may also be conducted under the auspices of the VA's Mental Health Strategic Healthcare Group (MHSHG), which supports the research efforts conducted at the National Center for PTSD, four Centers of Excellence (CoEs), and 10 Mental Illness Research Education and Clinical Centers (MIRECCs).[44]

The VA is currently partnering with the National Institute of Disability and Rehabilitation Research to develop the Traumatic Brain Injury Veterans Health Registry, which will facilitate future research by providing longitudinal data on the demographics, military service data, injury information, and treatment of all veterans with TBI.[45]

The Defense and Veterans Brain Injury Center (DVBIC), a component of the Defense Centers of Excellence for Psychological Health and Traumatic Brain Injury, is a collaboration between the VA and the DOD. Research conducted by the DVBIC includes randomized controlled trials of treatment strategies for TBI, epidemiologic studies of military-related TBI, and translational research involving brain imaging technology.[46]

Potential Issues for the 112th Congress

This part of the report focuses on ongoing issues that may be of interest to the 112th Congress, in the context of past congressional action addressing these issues. **Appendix C** summarizes provisions of public laws that address TBI among veterans, beginning with the 108th Congress and ending with the 111th Congress. In addition to specific issues noted here, a number of initiatives are in the planning and implementation process, providing opportunities for Congress to exercise its oversight function while programs are implemented and research is conducted.

Ongoing Issues in Access to Care

By extending the period of enhanced eligibility for OEF/OIF veterans (as described in the text box, "Veterans Health Administration: Eligibility, Enrollment, and Services," above), the National Defense Authorization Act for Fiscal Year 2008 (P.L. 110-181) facilitated access to care. However, a veteran's own behavior—whether intentional or not—may interfere with his or her ability to access the VA health care system and thus be properly diagnosed. Some veterans may choose not to disclose symptoms of TBI because they believe that being diagnosed with a TBI would affect their ability to stay in the National Guard or Reserves, or affect other future employment plans.[47] Similarly, some servicemembers leaving war zones may not disclose mental health symptoms, or may downplay such symptoms, in order to avoid any delay in their return home.[48] Some veterans may not be fully aware of changes in their functioning due to TBI.[49] Cognitive impairments due to TBI may compromise veterans' ability to seek care or navigate the system.[50]

Ongoing Issues in Identification of TBI

In addition to facilitating access to care (as noted above), P.L. 110-181 contributed to the identification of TBI by directing the Secretaries of the VA and DOD to propose medical codes to indicate TBI on medical records; this law also contributed to identification of TBI by requiring the VA Secretary to establish and maintain a TBI Veterans Health Registry. The Traumatic Brain Injury Act of 2008 (P.L. 110-206) also contributed to identification of TBI by involving HHS in tracking the incidence and prevalence of TBI among veterans. Ongoing issues in identification of TBI among OEF/OIF veterans at VA medical facilities generally fall into two categories—the screening instrument and how it is used.

Because the VA modified an existing screening instrument, the VA is responsible for establishing its validity and reliability for use with a slightly different population (i.e., OEF/OIF veterans receiving care from the VA, rather than servicemembers returning from OEF/OIF). Clinical validity refers to both how well the screening instrument identifies patients with TBI (i.e., sensitivity) and how well it identifies patients without TBI (i.e., specificity). At least one study has found that the screening instrument has high sensitivity and moderate specificity.[51] Because a positive screen is followed by a more thorough evaluation, sensitivity is more important than specificity in the screening instrument.

Reliability is the ability of the screening instrument to yield the same results if administered repeatedly to the same person. A small, preliminary study of test-retest reliability found that most items in the screening instrument do not have good reliability.[52] A larger study found that the screening instrument has high test-retest reliability.[53] Another VA study is in progress.[54]

The VA is also responsible for ensuring that the screening instrument is used as intended, by properly trained staff. Investigations have found that some providers used the screening instrument before being trained,[55] and that some OEF/OIF veterans were not screened or had delayed screenings because staff were not aware of procedures.[56] The VA is currently tracking completion and timeliness of TBI screenings and follow-up evaluations at the VISN level.[57]

Ongoing Issues in Treatment of TBI

Several laws have addressed treatment of TBI provided by either professionals or family caregivers. The Veterans Health Programs Improvement Act of 2004 (P.L. 108-422) resulted in the establishment of the Polytrauma System of Care. The Caregivers and Veterans Omnibus Health Services Act of 2010 (P.L. 111-163) built on work initiated under the National Defense Authorization Act for Fiscal Year 2007 (P.L. 109-364) in training family caregivers for veterans; P.L. 111-163 also enabled the VA to utilize non-VA facilities under certain circumstances.

An ongoing issue in treatment of TBI is coordination of care. Programs intended to improve coordination of care between VA and DOD may face their own coordination challenges. A 2011 report by the GAO identified challenges the Federal Recovery Coordinator Program is facing, including in coordination with other programs.[58] Because the majority of enrollees are enrolled in at least one other program for wounded servicemembers or veterans, the program must coordinate not only among care providers, but also among other care coordinators. Having multiple care coordinators increases the potential for duplication of effort, conflicting treatment goals, or failure to address issues (if each coordinator thinks someone else is handling the issue).

Ongoing Issues in TBI Research

Congress has appropriated funds for many research projects related to TBI. For example, the National Defense Authorization Act for Fiscal Year 2008 (P.L. 110-181) required the VA to collaborate with the TBI rehabilitation research community, grantees of the National Institute of Disability and Rehabilitation Research (within the Department of Education), the Defense and Veterans Brain Injury Center, and other governmental entities engaged in TBI rehabilitation.

The large number of studies conducted by the VA, DOD, and HHS (including both the Centers for Disease Control and Prevention and the National Institutes of Health) raises questions for some about potential duplication of effort, gaps in the research, dissemination of research findings, and translation of research into practice. While duplication of effort may seem wasteful, replicating studies is a normal part of the research process; ideally, the replicated studies yield the same results as the original study and thus increase confidence in the findings. The direction of subsequent research is often guided by identifying gaps in the existing research. Dissemination of research findings is necessary in order for the findings to be useful, and strong findings should be translated into practice in order to improve care.

APPENDIX A. OEF/OIF VETERANS WITH TBI, BY STATE

Table A-1. Number of OEF/OIFVeterans Diagnosed with TBI-Related Conditions at VA Medical Facilities, FY2002-FY2010, by State of Residence

Alabama	766	Nevada	286
Alaska	258	New Hampshire	232
Arizona	1,049	New Jersey	480
Arkansas	1,106	New Mexico	292
California	5,084	New York	1,934
Colorado	1,158	North Carolina	1,842
Connecticut	280	North Dakota	219
Delaware	91	Ohio	1,389
District Of Columbia	93	Oklahoma	1,203
Florida	2,383	Oregon	706
Georgia	1,725	Pennsylvania	1,350
Hawaii	361	Rhode Island	129
Idaho	244	South Carolina	379
Illinois	1,116	South Dakota	224
Indiana	816	Tennessee	1,017
Iowa	369	Texas	4,075
Kansas	693	Utah	221
Kentucky	1,243	Vermont	163
Louisiana	505	Virginia	1,050
Maine	185	Washington	1,645
Maryland	493	West Virginia	256
Massachusetts	636	Wisconsin	704
Michigan	790	Wyoming	147
Minnesota	1,028		
Mississippi	331	Puerto Rico	459
Missouri	796	Other	577
Montana	363	Unknown	336

Source: Response to CRS inquiry to VA Program Office, December 23, 2010.

Notes: Status as an OEF/OIF veteran is based on OEF/OIF deployment rosters from the DOD Defense Manpower Data Center with the last out-of-country dates through August 2010. Diagnoses were made during outpatient visits and hospitalizations at VA medical facilities between FY2002Q1 and FY2010Q4. TBI-related conditions are defined by VA Environmental Epidemiology System as the following ICD-9-CM codes: 310.2, 800, 801, 802, 803, 804, 850, 851, 852, 853, 854, 950. Each veteran may be diagnosed in the VA medical system with multiple TBI-related conditions, but is counted only once in the table. State of residence taken from first record of deployment in support of OEF/OIF. Due to the duration of OEF/OIF and repeated deployments, a number of the veterans who died in-theater may have previously accessed VA health care services and may therefore be included in these counts.

APPENDIX B. FLOWCHART OF VA PROCESS FOR IDENTIFYING AND TREATING TBI

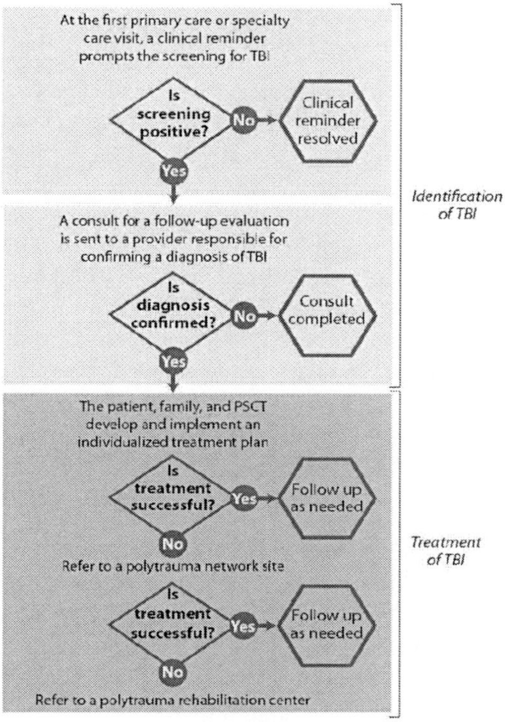

Source: Visual depiction of the identification and treatment processes described under the heading "TBI Among Veterans."

Notes: VA = Department of Veterans Affairs; TBI = Traumatic Brain Injury; PSCT = Polytrauma Support Clinic Team.

Figure B-1. Flowchart of VA Process for Identifying and Treating TBI.

APPENDIX C. PAST CONGRESSIONAL ACTION

Table C-1 summarizes provisions of public laws that address TBI among veterans, beginning with the 108th Congress and ending with the 111th Congress. Note that many of the laws listed in **Table C-1** do not focus on the VA, but include provisions relevant to veterans. For example, the National Defense Authorization Act for Fiscal Year 2007 (P.L. 109-364) primarily addresses the DOD, but is included because the panel it requires the DOD Secretary to establish is responsible for developing curricula for training family members in the provision of care and assistance to veterans (and servicemembers) with TBI. Similarly, the Traumatic Brain Injury Act of 2008 (P.L. 110-206) primarily addresses HHS, but is included because of a requirement that the HHS Secretary report on activities and procedures that can be implemented by the Centers for Disease Control and Prevention (CDC) to improve the collection and dissemination of epidemiological studies on the incidence and prevalence of TBI in veterans.

Table C-1. Congressional Action onTBI AmongVeterans, 2004-2010 (Excludes provisions focused on servicemembers, rather than veterans)

Public Law	Short Title	Key Provisions Related to TBI Among Veterans
P.L. 108-422	Veterans Health Programs Improvement Act of 2004	Directs the VA to designate an appropriate number of cooperative centers for clinical care, consultation, research, and education activities on polytrauma (i.e., the Polytrauma System of Care).
P.L. 109-364	John Warner National Defense Authorization Act for Fiscal Year 2007	Requires the DOD Secretary to establish a Traumatic Brain Injury Family Caregiver Panel to develop curricula for training family members in the provision of care and assistance to servicemembers and veterans with TBI.
P.L. 110-161	Consolidated Appropriations Act, 2008	Authorizes the VA Secretary to transfer up to $5 million to the HHS Secretary for the Graduate Psychology Education Program to support increased training of psychologists in the treatment of TBI, PTSD, and related disorders. [Same provision appears in P.L. 110-329 and P.L. 111-117.]
P.L. 110-181	National Defense Authorization Act for Fiscal Year 2008	Extends the period of enhanced eligibility for OEF/OIF veterans. Directs the VA and DOD Secretaries to propose codes for inclusion in the ICD to ensure that veterans and servicemembers with TBI receive a medical designation concomitant with the injury. Requires the VA Secretary, in selecting locations for an assisted-living services pilot program, to give special consideration to rural areas and locations with a high concentration of TBI. Requires the VA Secretary to establish and maintain a TBI Veterans Health Registry, including information about each OEF/OIF veteran who exhibits symptoms associated with TBI and applies for care or files a claim for disability compensation from VA. The VA is to notify veterans in the registry of significant developments in research on health consequences of OEF/OIF service. Requires the VA to collaborate with the TBI rehabilitation research community, grantees of the NIDRR of the Department of Education, the DVBIC, and other governmental entities engaged in TBI rehabilitation.
P.L. 110-206	Traumatic Brain Injury Act of 2008	Requires the HHS Secretary to report on activities and procedures that can be implemented by the CDC to improve the collection and dissemination of compatible epidemiological studies on the incidence and prevalence of TBI in veterans.
P.L. 110-329	Consolidated Security, Disaster Assistance, and Continuing	Authorizes the VA Secretary to transfer up to $5 million to the HHS Secretary for the Graduate Psychology Education Program to support increased training of psychologists in the treatment of TBI, PTSD, and related disorders.

Public Law	Short Title	Key Provisions Related to TBI Among Veterans
	Appropriations Act, 2009	[Same provision appears in P.L. 110-161 and P.L. 111-117.]
P.L. 111-117	Consolidated Appropriations Act, 2010	Authorizes the VA Secretary to transfer up to $5 million to the HHS Secretary for the Graduate Psychology Education Program to support increased training of psychologists in the treatment of TBI, PTSD, and related disorders. [Same provision appears in P.L. 110-161 and P.L. 110-329.]
P.L. 111-163	Caregivers and Veterans Omnibus Health Services Act of 2010	Directs the VA Secretary to establish a program of comprehensive assistance for family caregivers of eligible veterans, including those with TBI. Once fully implemented, the program will include instruction and training in personal care services; ongoing technical support; counseling; and lodging and subsistence while accompanying the veteran for VA medical care. The program will also allow additional assistance for the primary personal care provider, including mental health services, respite care, and a monthly stipend comparable to that provided to commercial caregivers in that geographic area. Authorizes the VA Secretary to utilize non-VA facilities (that meet accreditation standards) for the care and treatment of veterans with TBI, and to contract with non-VA providers for specialized residential care and rehabilitation services to veterans with TBI who would otherwise require nursing home admission. Directs the VA Secretary to establish the Committee on Care of Veterans with TBI, to continually assess VA capabilities to meet the treatment and rehabilitation needs of veterans with TBI.

Source: CRS analysis of data from the Legislative Information Service.

Notes: TBI = Traumatic Brain Injury; OEF/OIF = Operation Enduring Freedom and Operation Iraqi Freedom (including Operation New Dawn); VA = Department of Veterans Affairs; DOD = Department of Defense; HHS = Department of Health and Human Services; CDC = Centers for Disease Control and Prevention; ICD = International Classification of Diseases; DVBIC = Defense and Veterans Brain Injury Center; NIDRR = National Institute of Disability and Rehabilitation Research.

End Notes

[1] Operation Enduring Freedom (OEF) began on October 7, 2001, and continues today. Operation Iraqi Freedom (OIF) began on March 20, 2003; on September 1, 2010, OIF was redesignated Operation New Dawn, which continues today. (These operations are not defined in statute; the dates presented here are commonly accepted.) The abbreviation OEF/OIF is used throughout this report to refer to Operation Enduring Freedom and Operation Iraqi Freedom (now called Operation New Dawn).

[2] This report focuses on TBI as a health care issue, and therefore does not address classification of TBI as a service-connected disability for compensation purposes; for a general discussion of veterans' disability benefits, refer to CRS Report RL34626, *Veterans' Benefits: Benefits Available for Disabled Veterans*, by Christine Scott and Carol D. Davis. This report does not address TBI in the military health care system, except where necessary to provide context or explain joint endeavors of the Departments of Defense and Veterans Affairs; for information about the military health care system, refer to CRS Report RL33537, *Military Medical Care: Questions and Answers*, by Don J. Jansen. For information about TBI among professional football players,

refer to CRS Report R41555, *NFL Players and Efforts to Protect Them From Concussions*, by L. Elaine Halchin.

[3] Brain Injury Association of America, "BIAA Adopts New TBI Definition," press release, February 6, 2011,http://www.biausa.org/AnnouncementRetrieve.aspx?ID=66290.

[4] Mark Faul, Likang Xu, and Marlena M. Wald, et al., *Traumatic Brain Injury in the United States: Emergency Department Visits, Hospitalizations, and Deaths*, Centers for Disease Control and Prevention, National Center forInjury Prevention and Control, Atlanta, GA, March 2010, http://www.cdc.gov/traumaticbraininjury/pdf/blue_book.pdf.

[5] Terri Tanielian and Lisa H. Jaycox, eds. *Invisible Wounds of War: Psychological and Cognitive Injuries, Their Consequences, and Services to Assist Recovery*, RAND Corporation, 2008, p. 310, http://www.rand.org/pubs/monographs/2008/RAND_MG720.pdf.

[6] Defense and Veterans Brain Injury Center, *DOD Numbers for Traumatic Brain Injury*, http://www.dvbic.org/TBI-Numbers.aspx.

[7] Marcia Vital, *Traumatic Brain Injury: Hope Through Research*, National Institutes of Health, National Institute of Neurological Disorders and Stroke, NIH Publication No. 02-158, Bethesda, MD, September 2002,http://www.ninds.nih.gov/disorders/tbi/tbi_htr.pdf.

[8] Michael S. Jaffee, Kathy M. Helmick, and Philip D. Girard, et al., "Acute clinical care and care coordination within Department of Defense," *Journal of Rehabilitation Research & Development*, vol. 46, no. 6 (2009), pp. 655-666.

[9] Marcia Vital, *Traumatic Brain Injury: Hope Through Research*, National Institutes of Health, National Institute of Neurological Disorders and Stroke, NIH Publication No. 02-158, Bethesda, MD, September 2002 http://www.ninds.nih.gov/ disorders/tbi/tbi_htr.pdf.

[10] Marcia Vital, *Traumatic Brain Injury: Hope Through Research*, National Institutes of Health, National Institute of Neurological Disorders and Stroke, NIH Publication No. 02-158, Bethesda, MD, September 2002, http://www.ninds.nih.gov/ disorders/tbi/tbi_htr.pdf.

[11] Ibid.

[12] Brent E. Masel and Douglas S. DeWitt, "Traumatic Brain Injury: A Disease Process, Not an Event," *Journal of Neurotrauma*, no. 27 (August 2010), p. 1529–1540; and Terri Tanielian and Lisa H. Jaycox, eds. *Invisible Wounds of War: Psychological and Cognitive Injuries, Their Consequences, and Services to Assist Recovery*, RAND Corporation, 2008, p. 310, http://www.rand.org/pubs/monographs/2008/RAND_MG720.pdf.

[13] Brent E. Masel and Douglas S. DeWitt, "Traumatic Brain Injury: A Disease Process, Not an Event," *Journal of Neurotrauma*, no. 27 (August 2010), p. 1529–1540; and Institute of Medicine (IOM), *Gulf War and Health, Volume 7: Long-term Consequences of Traumatic Brain Injury* (Washington, DC: The National Academies Press, 2009).

[14] Ibid.

[15] Geoffrey Ling, Faris Bandak, and Rocco Armonda, et al., "Explosive Blast Neurotrauma," *Journal of Neutrotrauma*, vol. 26 (2009), pp. 815-825.

[16] Atul Gawande, "Casualties of War—Military Care for the Wounded from Iraq and Afghanistan," *New England Journal of Medicine*, vol. 351, no. 24 (2004), pp. 2471-2475.

[17] Office of the Surgeon General, Center for Excellence in Medical Multimedia, *Traumatic Brain Injury: The Journey Home*, http://www.traumaticbraininjuryatoz.org.

[18] Terri Tanielian and Lisa H. Jaycox, eds. *Invisible Wounds of War: Psychological and Cognitive Injuries, Their Consequences, and Services to Assist Recovery*, RAND Corporation, 2008, p. 47, http://www.rand.org/pubs/monographs/2008/RAND_MG720.pdf.

[19] U.S. Department of Veterans Affairs, Office of Public Health and Environmental Hazards, Analysis of VA Health Care Utilization among Operation Enduring Freedom (OEF) and Operation Iraqi Freedom (OIF) Veterans, Cumulative from 1st Quarter FY2002 through 4th Quarter FY2010, December 2010.

[20] Response to CRS inquiry to VA Program Office, December 23, 2010.

[21] Department of Veterans Affairs, *Letter to OEF/OIF Veterans*, http://www.gibill.va.gov/documents/CH33_veteran_outreach_letter.pdf.

[22] Department of Veterans Affairs, *Returning Service Members (OEF/OIF): Welcome Home and Outreach*, http://www.oefoif.va.gov/WelcomeHomeOutreach.asp.

[23] Department of Veterans Affairs, Public and Intergovernmental Affairs, *VA Video Outreach Message Aimed at New Veterans*, http://www1.va.gov/opa/pressrel/pressrelease.cfm?id= 1981.

[24] The DOD Yellow Ribbon Program, established under the National Defense Authorization Act for Fiscal Year 2008, enacted 1/28/2008 (P.L. 110-181), is distinct from the VA Yellow Ribbon Program (which focuses on education).

[25] Department of Veterans Affairs, *Returning Service Members (OEF/OIF): Seven Touches of Outreach*, http://www.oefoif.va.gov/SevenTouchesOutreach.asp.

[26] U.S. Department of Veterans Affairs, Office of Public Health and Environmental Hazards, Analysis of VA Health Care Utilization among Operation Enduring Freedom (OEF) and Operation Iraqi Freedom (OIF) Veterans, Cumulative from 1st Quarter FY2002 through 4th Quarter FY2010, December 2010.

[27] TRICARE is a system of military and private health care offering benefits for active duty servicemembers, National Guard and Reserve members, military retirees, their families, survivors, and certain former spouses. See CRS Report RL33537, *Military Medical Care: Questions and Answers*, by Don J. Jansen.

[28] Department of Veterans Affairs, Veterans Health Administration, Screening and Evaluation of Possible Traumatic Brain Injury in Operation Enduring Freedom (OEF) and Operation Iraqi Freedom (OIF) Veterans, VHA Directive 2007-013, April 13, 2007; unless otherwise noted, all information in this subsection is drawn from this source.

[29] This reminder, together with reminders for screens for PTSD, depression, alcohol abuse, and infectious diseases endemic to Southwest Asia, constitutes the "Afghan and Iraq Post-Deployment Screen." Veterans Health Administration, *Implementation of the National Clinical Reminder for Afghan and Iraq Post-Deployment Screening*, Department of Veterans Affairs, VHA Directive 2005-055, Washington, DC, December 1, 2005.

[30] Posttraumatic stress disorder (PTSD) is an anxiety disorder that may occur following a traumatic event.

[31] American Psychiatric Association, *Diagnostic and Statistical Manual of Mental Disorders*, Fourth Edition, Text Revision (Arlington, VA: American Psychiatric Association, 2000), pp. 463-468.

[32] The VA is studying differential diagnoses, in an effort to build objective and consistent diagnostic criteria for TBI and PTSD. Department of Veterans Affairs, Office of Public Health and Environmental Hazards, http://www.publichealth.va.gov/research/epidemiology.

[33] Department of Veterans Affairs, Veterans Health Administration, Screening and Evaluation of Possible Traumatic Brain Injury in Operation Enduring Freedom (OEF) and Operation Iraqi Freedom (OIF) Veterans, VHA Directive 2007-013, April 13, 2007.

[34] Response to CRS inquiry to VA Program Office, January 5, 2011.

[35] Mild TBI accounted for 81% of the servicemembers sustaining TBI in 2010. Defense and Veterans Brain Injury Center, *DOD Numbers for Traumatic Brain Injury*, http://www.dvbic. org/TBI-Numbers.aspx.

[36] Charles W. Hoge, Dennis McGurk, and Jeffrey L. Thomas et al., "Mild Traumatic Brain Injury in US Soldiers Returning from Iraq," *New England Journal of Medicine*, vol. 358, no. 5 (2008), pp. 453-463.

[37] Department of Veterans Affairs and Department of Defense, *VA/DOD Clinical Practice Guideline for Management of Concussion/mild Traumatic Brain Injury (mTBI)*, April 2009, http://www.healthquality. va.gov/management_of_concussion_mtbi.asp.

[38] Veterans Health Administration, *Polytrauma-Traumatic Brain Injury (TBI) System of Care*, Department of Veterans Affairs, VHA Directive 2009-028, Washington, DC, June 9, 2009; unless otherwise noted, all information in this subsection is drawn from this source. Polytrauma is defined therein as "two or more injuries sustained in the same incident that affect multiple body parts or organ systems and result in physical cognitive, psychological, or psychosocial impairments and functional disabilities."

[39] Department of Veterans Affairs, Returning Service Members *(OEF/OIF)*, http://www.oefoif. va.gov.

[40] U.S. Congress, House Committee on Veterans' Affairs, Subcommittee on Oversight and Investigations, *Leaving No One Behind: Is the Federal Recovery Coordination Program Working?* 111th Cong., 1st sess., April 28, 2009, Opening Statement of Chairman Mitchell.

[41] Department of Veterans Affairs, *Congressional Submission: FY 2011 Funding and FY 2012 Advance Appropriations Request*, http://www.va.gov/budget/docs/summary/Fy2012 _Volume_I-Summary_Volume. pdf.

[42] Department of Defense and Full-Year Continuing Appropriations Act, 2011, enacted April 15, 2011 (P.L. 112-10).

[43] Department of Veterans Affairs, Office of Research and Development, *Program Announcement: Traumatic Brain Injury*, June 17, 2008.

[44] U.S. Department of Veterans Affairs, *MIRECCs and Centers of Excellence*, http://www. mirecc.va.gov/national-mirecc-overview.asp.

[45] Department of Veterans Affairs, *Two VA Initiatives on Traumatic Brain Injury in Veterans*, March 2010, http://www.publichealth.va.gov/docs/epidemiology/TBI_brochure.pdf.

[46] Defense and Veterans Brain Injury Center, *Research*, http://www.dvbic.org/Research.aspx.

[47] U.S. Government Accountability Office, Mild Traumatic Brain Injury Screening and Evaluation Implemented for OEF/OIF Veterans, but Challenges Remain, 08-276, February 2008.

[48] Terri Tanielian and Lisa H. Jaycox, eds. *Invisible Wounds of War: Psychological and Cognitive Injuries, Their Consequences, and Services to Assist Recovery*, RAND Corporation, 2008, p. 7, http://www.rand.org/pubs/ monographs/2008/RAND_MG720.pdf.

[49] Rodney D. Vanderploeg, Heather G. Belanger, and Jennifer D. Duchnick et al., "Awareness Problems Following Moderate to Severe Traumatic Brain Injury: Prevalence, Assessment Methods, and Injury Correlates," *Journal of Rehabilitation Research & Development*, vol. 44, no. 7 (2007), pp. 937-950.

[50] Henry L. Lew, John H. Poole, and Sylvia B. Guillory et al., "Persistent Problems after Traumatic Brain Injury: The Need for Long-Term Follow-up and Coordinated Care," *Journal of Rehabilitation Research & Development*, vol. 43 (2006), pp. vii-x.

[51] K.T. Donnelly, J.P. Donnelly, and M. Dunnamm, et al., "Reliability, Sensitivity, and Specificity of the VA Traumatic Brain Injury Screening Tool," *Journal of Head Trauma Rehabilitation*, E-pub ahead of print 2011.

[52] Sarah A. Van Dyke, Bradley N. Axelrod, and Christian Schutte, "Test-Retest Reliability of the Traumatic Brain Injury Screening Instrument," *Military Medicine*, vol. 175, no. 12 (2010), pp. 947-949.

[53] K.T. Donnelly, J.P. Donnelly, and M. Dunnamm, et al., "Reliability, Sensitivity, and Specificity of the VA Traumatic Brain Injury Screening Tool," *Journal of Head Trauma Rehabilitation*, Epub ahead of print 2011.

[54] Department of Veterans Affairs (Babcock-Parziale, Judi - Principal Investigator), *Evaluation of VA's TBI Clinical Reminder And Secondary Level Evaluation*, ClinicalTrials.gov Identifier: NCT00852527, http://clinical trials.gov/ ct2/ show/NCT00852527.

[55] U.S. Government Accountability Office, VA Health Care: Mild Traumatic Brain Injury Screening and Evaluation Implemented for OEF/OIF Veterans, But Challenges Remain, GAO-08-276, February 2008, http://www. gao.gov.

[56] VA Office of Inspector General, Office of Audits & Evaluations, *Veterans Health Administration Audit of Community-Based Outpatient Clinic Management Oversight*, VAOIG-09-02093-211, July 28, 2010, http://www.va.gov/oig/52/reports/2010/VAOIG-09-02093-211.pdf.

[57] VA Quality Enhancement Research Initiative (QUERI), *Polytrauma/Blast-Related Injuries QUERI Center Strategic Plan*, December 2009, http://www.queri.research.va.gov/about/ strategic_plans/ptbri.pdf.

[58] U.S. Government Accountability Office, DOD and VA Health Care: Federal Recovery Coordination Program Continues to Expand but Faces Significant Challenges, GAO-11-250, March 23, 2011.

In: Veteran Injuries, Disorders and Medical Care Service
Editors: Jessica Michaels and Jesse E. Levine
ISBN: 978-1-62081-302-7

Chapter 5

SUICIDE PREVENTION EFFORTS OF THE VETERANS HEALTH ADMINISTRATION*

Erin Bagalman

SUMMARY

Responsibility for prevention of veteran suicide lies primarily with the Veterans Health Administration (VHA), within the Department of Veterans Affairs (VA). The VHA Strategic Plan for Suicide Prevention is based on a public health framework, which has three major components: (1) surveillance, (2) risk and protective factors, and (3) prevention interventions.

No nationwide surveillance system exists for suicide among all veterans; therefore, the actual incidence of suicide among veterans is not known. Surveillance, or systematic collection of data on completed (i.e., fatal) suicides, is essential to define the scope of the problem (i.e., the suicide rate among veterans), identify characteristics associated with higher or lower risk of suicide, and track changes in the suicide rate over time to evaluate suicide prevention interventions. In the absence of a nationwide surveillance system for veteran suicide, the VHA is attempting to determine the rate of suicide among veterans in two ways, both in collaboration with the Centers for Disease Control and Prevention (CDC).

Information collected in surveillance is used to identify suicide risk factors (i.e., characteristics associated with higher rates of suicide) and protective factors (i.e., characteristics associated with lower rates of suicide). This is essential in order to design interventions that reduce risk factors and/or increase protective factors, thus lowering overall risk of suicide. Risk factors are also helpful in identifying at-risk groups or individuals so that interventions can be delivered to the people who need them most. Within the VHA, this research is supported by the Office of Research and Development; a Center of Excellence in suicide prevention; and a Mental Illness Research, Education, and Clinical Center on suicide prevention.

The intervention cycle includes three stages: design and test interventions, implement interventions, and evaluate interventions. The research components mentioned above

* This is an edited, reformatted and augmented version of a Congressional Research Service publication, CRS Report *for Congress* R42340, *from* www.crs.gov, prepared for Members and Committees of Congress, *dated* February 3, 2012.

have roles in small-scale pilot testing and large-scale evaluations of interventions. This report discusses seven areas of VHA suicide prevention interventions: (1) easy access to care, (2) education, (3) screening and treatment, (4) limited access to lethal means, (5) suicide hotline, (6) media restrictions, and (7) suicide prevention coordinators.

This report identifies challenges the VHA faces in each component of suicide prevention and discusses potential issues for Congress. A recurring theme is the need for the VHA to work in concert with other federal, state, and local government agencies; private for-profit and not-forprofit health care providers; veterans, their families, and their communities; and other individuals or organizations that might be able to help. Specific challenges in surveillance include timeliness of data, accurate identification of decedents as veterans, and consistent classification of deaths as suicides. Challenges in risk and protective factors research include a need for more collaboration and dialogue among agencies involved in suicide prevention and across other areas of public health (because suicide has some of the same risk and protective factors as other public health problems). Challenges in VHA suicide prevention interventions also include the need for more collaboration and dialogue, as well as an apparent gap between policy and practice, and misperceptions about mental illness and mental health care.

INTRODUCTION

Congress has attempted to address the problem of suicide among veterans through legislation,[1] and the House and Senate Committees on Veterans' Affairs have conducted oversight hearings, both on prevention of veteran suicide specifically and on veteran mental health more broadly.[2] The actual number or rate of veteran suicides is not known, because no nationwide surveillance system for suicide among all veterans exists, but there is consensus that the number is too high.[3] Responsibility for prevention of veteran suicide lies primarily with the Veterans Health Administration (VHA), within the Department of Veterans Affairs (VA). Such a challenging task, however, demands collaboration with other federal agencies, state and local governments, other organizations, communities, and individuals.

Prevention of suicide can be approached in two ways, which are not mutually exclusive. The public health approach intervenes with populations (e.g., distributing educational materials about mental illness and mental health services), whereas the clinical approach intervenes with individuals (e.g., prescribing antidepressant medication to a person diagnosed with depression). The individual focus of the clinical approach limits its reach to those who access the health care system;[4] clinical interventions are necessary but not sufficient. If the goal is to reach a broader population, the public health approach is considered essential.

The public health approach provides the framework for two suicide prevention strategies that are referenced in this report. The National Strategy for Suicide Prevention[5] involves multiple federal departments, including the VA, Defense (DOD), and Education (ED), as well as several agencies within Health and Human Services (HHS).[6] The VHA Strategic Plan for Suicide Prevention[7] is a compilation of VHA activities related to suicide prevention. While this CRS report focuses on suicide prevention efforts of the VHA, activities of other entities are discussed as they relate to VHA activities.

The textbox briefly discusses eligibility for, enrollment in, and use of VHA services. As noted in the textbox, the majority of veterans do not use VHA services. VHA efforts to increase access to care—and to prevent suicide among veterans who do not use VHA services—are discussed later in this report.

Who Is a Veteran? Eligibility for, Enrollment in, and Use of VA Health Care

The term "veteran" may refer broadly to anyone who has served in the armed forces, including those currently serving. In this report, a veteran is someone who has separated from military service following a period of active duty. Although an individual may return to active duty following separation (a particular issue among National Guard and Reserve members who have been activated), current active duty servicemembers are not the focus of this report.

Three additional points may be made relative to veterans and VA health care services:

- *Eligibility:* Not all veterans are eligible for VA health care services (see http://www.va.gov/healthbenefits); Vet Centers (non-medical facilities that provide readjustment counseling services for veterans and their families) have their own eligibility criteria (see http://www.vetcenter. va.gov/Eligibility.asp).
- *Enrollment:* Not all eligible veterans enroll in VA health care services. The number of enrolled veterans in FY2010 was 8.3 million, which is 36.6% of the estimated veteran population of 22.7 million. As noted above, some veterans are not eligible for VA health care services; others may choose not to enroll for various reasons (e.g., they might have employer-sponsored health insurance or other sources of health care services).
- *Use:* Not all enrolled veterans actually use VA health care services. The number of veterans who received health care services in FY2010 was 5.4 million, which is 65.1% of the 8.3 million enrolled veterans, or 23.8% of the estimated veteran population of 22.7 million. Enrolled veterans may choose not to receive care for various reasons (e.g., they might not perceive a need for health care services).

Sources: Estimated number of veterans is from Department of Veterans Affairs, FY2012 Budget Submission, Summary Volume, Volume 1 of 4, February 2011, pp. 1F-1; numbers of veterans enrolled using services are from Department of Veterans Affairs, FY2012 Budget Submission, Medical Programs and Information Technology Programs, Volume 2 of 4, February 2011, pp. 1A-28. See also CRS Report R42324, "Who is a Veteran?"—Basic Eligibility for Veterans' Benefits, by Christine Scott.

The VHA has received both praise and criticism for its suicide prevention efforts and mental health services more generally. In 2010 the Suicide Prevention Resource Center, funded by the Substance Abuse and Mental Health Services Administration (SAMHSA), in collaboration with the non-profit Suicide Prevention Action Network, published a progress report on the National Strategy for Suicide Prevention; the progress report (hereinafter referred to as *Charting the Future*) praises VHA's suicide prevention practices and recommends disseminating them to the rest of the health care system.[8] *Charting the Future* describes the VHA as "one of the most vibrant forces in the U.S. suicide prevention movement, implementing multiple levels of innovation and state of the art interventions, backed up by a robust evaluation and research capacity."[9] In contrast, some congressional testimony has criticized VHA's suicide prevention efforts for inadequacies, such as barriers to accessing care and lack of evidence-based treatments for those who do access care.[10] A 2011 evaluation of VHA mental health services (not limited to suicide prevention efforts) by the Altarum Institute and RAND Health captures both sides of the argument, finding that VHA mental health care is generally at least as good as that of other health care systems, but that it "often does not meet implicit VA expectations."[11]

This report begins with a brief overview of the public health framework for suicide prevention. The three subsequent parts of the report correspond to the three major components of the public health framework: (1) suicide surveillance, (2) suicide risk factors and protective factors, and (3) suicide prevention interventions. The final section addresses potential issues for Congress.

The importance of collaboration and dialogue is a recurring theme across all components of the VHA's suicide prevention efforts. Surveillance requires collaboration to address timeliness of data, accurate identification of decedents as veterans, and consistent classification of deaths as suicides. Risk and protective factors research requires dialogue among agencies involved in suicide prevention and across other areas of public health (because suicide has some of the same risk and protective factors as other public health problems). Successful prevention interventions also require collaboration. Challenges in prevention interventions include an apparent gap between policy and practice, as well as misperceptions about mental illness and its treatment.

A PUBLIC HEALTH FRAMEWORK FOR SUICIDE PREVENTION

As noted previously, both the National Strategy for Suicide Prevention and the VHA Strategic Plan for Suicide Prevention are based on a public health framework. As illustrated in *Figure 1*, the framework has three major components: (1) surveillance, (2) risk and protective factors, and (3) prevention interventions. Suicide surveillance involves collecting data on completed (i.e., fatal) suicides in order to define the scope of the problem. Data collected in surveillance can be used to identify risk factors (i.e., characteristics associated with higher suicide risk) and protective factors (i.e., characteristics associated with lower suicide risk).

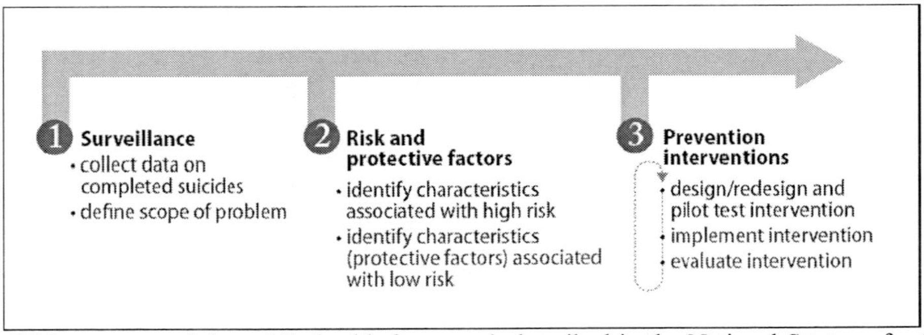

Source: CRS summary of the public health framework described in the National Strategy for Suicide Prevention. U.S. Department of Health and Human Services (HHS), Public Health Service, National Strategy for Suicide Prevention: Goals and Objectives for Action, SMA01-3517, Rockville, MD, 2001, http://store. samhsa.gov/product/ SMA01-3517, pp. 29-40.

Figure 1. A Public Health Framework for Suicide Prevention.

Suicide prevention interventions aim to reduce risk factors and/or enhance protective factors that have been identified; interventions may target high-risk groups or individuals, identified based on known risk factors.

SUICIDE SURVEILLANCE

As noted previously, no nationwide surveillance system exists for suicide among all veterans. Surveillance, or systematic collection of data on completed (i.e., fatal) suicides, is essential for three purposes. First, surveillance defines the scope of the problem, i.e., the suicide rate among veterans. Second, information from surveillance is used to identify characteristics associated with higher or lower risk of suicide. Third, information from surveillance is used to track changes in the suicide rate over time and evaluate suicide prevention interventions. In order to evaluate interventions, suicide surveillance must measure the same thing, in the same way, repeatedly over time.

In the absence of a nationwide surveillance system for veteran suicide, the VHA is attempting to determine the rate of suicide among veterans in two ways, both in collaboration with the Centers for Disease Control and Prevention (CDC). Combining the two methods provides more information about veteran suicide than either method alone, but the combination remains inadequate to the task. For example, one method is limited to enrolled veterans, and the other is limited to fewer than half the states; thus even the combination does not capture all veteran suicides. Also, statistics from both methods have a lag time of years, so that timeliness of data is an ongoing challenge. Each of the two methods is described below, along with its limitations and (where applicable) efforts to overcome those limitations.

Combining VHA Data with the National Death Index (NDI)

The VHA's primary approach to surveillance is illustrated in *Figure 2.* Information about completed (i.e., fatal) suicides is collected in death certificates by state, territorial, and local governments;[12] aggregated into the National Death Index (NDI) by the CDC;[13] and combined with enrollment data by the VHA in order to identify suicides among enrolled veterans.[14]

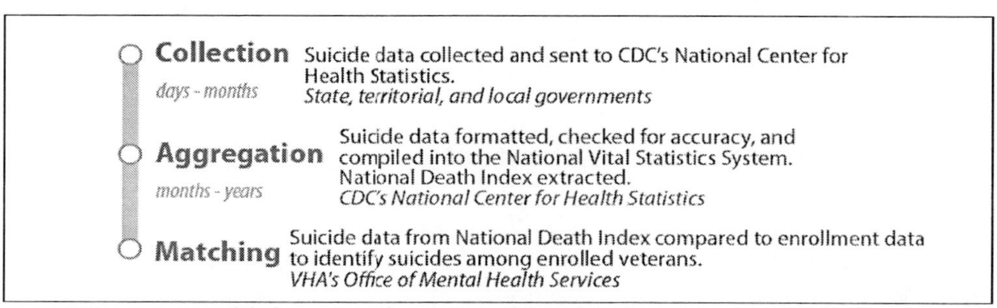

Source: CRS summary of information from CDC, National Center for Health Statistics, About the National Death Index, http://www.cdc.gov/nchs/data_ access /ndi/about_ndi.htm; and from the VHA.

Figure 2. Combining VHA Data with the National Death Index.

This approach is subject to the following limitations:

- The resulting data may not be comparable across jurisdictions.[15]
- The lag between a suicide event and identification of the decedent as an enrolled veteran may be years; this delays the availability of crucial information.
- Suicides among non-enrolled veterans are not captured;[16] this leaves out the majority of veterans.[17]

Accessing the National Violent Death Reporting System (NVDRS)

In an attempt to identify suicides among veterans regardless of enrollment with the VA, the VHA uses the CDC's National Violent Death Reporting System (NVDRS), among other sources of information.18 The NVDRS is a CDC-funded program that enables participating states to supplement death certificates with information from law enforcement agencies, crime laboratories, coroner or medical examiner reports, health providers, and other state and local agencies. Through ongoing active surveillance, NVDRS may increase the likelihood that a death is recognized as a suicide and that a decedent's veteran status is captured (regardless of enrollment with the VHA). The CDC is working to address the limitations of this approach through the following activities:

- Expand the NVDRS to all 50 states, the District of Columbia, and the territories;[19] currently, the NVDRS is in operation in fewer than half the states.[20]
- Increase standardization of data collection and analysis, in order to increase comparability across states.[21]
- Assess the feasibility of linking VHA data directly to state NVDRS programs, thereby eliminating a step in the process and potentially reducing the lag time.[22]
- Link the NVDRS to data from the VHA and the DOD's Suicide Event Report, in order to increase accurate identification of veteran status.[23]

The timeliness of the data is a challenge for the VHA in both methods of surveillance described above. This is a challenge for suicide surveillance nationwide, not limited to suicide surveillance among veterans. Timely reporting of death certificates is identified as a core issue in the 2010 update to the National Strategy for Suicide Prevention.[24]

Suicide Risk Factors and Protective Factors

Identifying characteristics associated with higher rates of suicide (i.e., risk factors) and lower rates of suicide (i.e., protective factors) is essential in order to design effective interventions. Suicide prevention interventions aim to reduce risk factors and/or increase protective factors, thus lowering overall risk of suicide. Knowing what the risk factors are also helps in identifying at-risk groups or individuals so that interventions can be delivered to the people who need them most. Thus the second step in the public health framework for suicide prevention is identification of suicide risk and protective factors using data collected in surveillance. *Table 1* provides examples of risk and protective factors among the general population.

Table 1. Selected Risk and Protective Factors in the General Population

Risk Factors	Protective Factors
Some major physical illnesses, mental disorders, and substance use disorders	Effective clinical care for physical illnesses, mental disorders, and substance use disorders
Barriers to accessing health care	Easy access to a variety of clinical interventions
Stigma associated with help-seeking behavior	Support for help-seeking behavior
Easy access to lethal means (e.g., firearms or poison)	Restricted access to lethal means (e.g., firearms or poison)
Lack of social support and sense of isolation	Strong connections to family and community support
Cultural/religious beliefs that accept suicide	Cultural/religious beliefs that discourage suicide

Source: Examples of risk and protective factors selected from U.S. Department of Health and Human Services (HHS), Public Health Service, National Strategy for Suicide Prevention: Goals and Objectives for Action, SMA01-3517, Rockville, MD, 2001, pp. 35-36, http://store.samhsa.gov/product/SMA01-3517.

Veteran-specific research on suicide risk and protective factors is necessary, because the veteran population differs from the non-veteran population on a variety of characteristics (e.g., gender distribution), some of which may also be associated with suicide risk. The subpopulation of veterans who are enrolled with the VHA may differ from non-enrolled veterans, as well.

The VHA conducts veteran-specific research that builds on research among the general population. Within HHS, both the CDC[25] and the National Institute of Mental Health (NIMH)[26] disseminate research on suicide risk and protective factors within the general population. Also, SAMHSA collects data on suicide attempts and related behavior.[27]

It should be noted that risk factors for attempted suicide may differ from risk factors for completed suicide; for example, women have a higher rate of attempted suicide, but men have a higher rate of completed suicide.[28] Despite a large number of risk and protective factors identified by researchers, it is not yet possible to predict who will attempt or complete suicide.[29] The inability to identify individuals most in need of interventions is one of the reasons a public health approach—with a focus on population-level interventions—is necessary for effective suicide prevention.

Within the VHA, mental health research—including research on suicide risk and protective factors—is supported by two organizational units: the Office of Research and Development (ORD) and the Mental Health Strategic Healthcare Group (MHSHG). In general, the ORD funds intramural research by individual VHA investigators or researchers (including mental health care research).[30]

The MHSHG funds a Center of Excellence (COE) in suicide prevention and a Mental Illness Research, Education, and Clinical Center (MIRECC) on suicide prevention, as well as centers addressing other mental health topics. Examples of research conducted on risk and protective factors by each of these three components—ORD, COE, and MIRECC—are provided below.

The same three research components are also involved in the development and evaluation of suicide prevention interventions.

VHA Office of Research and Development (ORD)

The ORD's Health Services Research and Development Service supports research into suicide risk factors and protective factors.[31]

For example, the VHA conducted a study to identify patient characteristics associated with higher suicide rates among veterans in treatment for depression (a known risk factor in the general population, as well as among veterans).[32]

Another study examined characteristics associated with suicide risk among patients seen in VHA primary care, to help identify factors that primary care providers may be able to use to detect suicide risk.[33] These studies, and others like them, can help the VHA identify veterans at high risk of suicide, so that interventions can be targeted to them.

Center of Excellence (COE)

The COE at Canandaigua, New York, conducts research on suicide risk factors and protective factors, in addition to other suicide prevention activities. Established in August 2007 at the direction of Congress,[34] the COE has the mission of developing and studying evidence-based public health approaches to prevention of veteran suicide, with the goal of reducing morbidity and mortality associated with suicide in the veteran population. In pursuit of its mission, the Epidemiology and Interventions Research Core within the COE collects and analyzes data on suicide risk factors and protective factors (as well as other topics) among both veterans who use VHA services and those who do not.[35]

Mental Illness Research, Education, and Clinical Center (MIRECC)

The MIRECCs, also established at the direction of Congress,[36] conduct research on a range of mental health-related topics, including suicide risk factors and protective factors. Specifically, the MIRECC of the VA Rocky Mountain Network pursues the goal of reducing suicidality in the veteran population, by conducting research on potential contributions of cognitive and neurobiological factors, among other activities.[37]

For example, one study assesses the relationship (if any) between prolonged grief and suicidal ideation.[38] Another study investigates the neurobiology of suicide risk in traumatic brain injury and substance abuse.[39] Other MIRECCs may also conduct research related to suicide, in the course of pursuing their other goals.

Suicide Prevention Interventions

Through effective suicide prevention interventions, people's lives can be saved. Interventions aim to reduce risk factors and/or enhance protective factors, thereby lowering the risk of suicide. They may address entire populations (e.g., all veterans), at-risk subgroups (e.g., veterans diagnosed with PTSD), or high-risk individuals (e.g., veterans with recent suicide attempts).

Suicide prevention interventions are refined in a three-stage cycle. The first stage is to develop and pilot test interventions on a small scale to ensure that they are safe, ethical, feasible, efficacious (i.e., they work under ideal conditions), and effective (i.e., they work under real-world conditions). If interventions are successful in the first stage, the second stage is to implement them on a larger scale. The third stage is to evaluate interventions that have been implemented on a larger scale, to verify their effectiveness and determine for whom they are most effective. The three stages can then be repeated to refine interventions, either to improve their effectiveness or to adjust them for use with a different population (e.g., applying an intervention developed for male veterans to a population of female veterans).

Within the VHA, the same three research components involved in risk and protective factors research are involved in the intervention cycle: ORD,[40] COE,[41] and MIRECC.[42] Because small-scale testing and large-scale evaluation are both integral to suicide prevention interventions, it is worth noting that rigorous research on effectiveness is difficult and lacking for most interventions, both within and outside the VHA.[43]

The rest of this section discusses seven areas of VHA suicide prevention interventions: (1) easy access to care, (2) education, (3) screening and treatment, (4) limited access to lethal means, (5) suicide hotline, (6) media restrictions, and (7) suicide prevention coordinators.

Easy Access to Care

As noted previously, the majority of veterans do not use VHA services. Easy access to care is a protective factor against suicide,[44] and the VHA is making efforts to increase access to care by addressing identified barriers to care, including logistical challenges in scheduling or attending appointments, lack of understanding or awareness of mental health care, stigma associated with mental illness, and concerns about VHA care. In order to address these barriers, the VHA is taking two broad approaches: (1) increasing access to care by offering a broader range of mental health services (e.g., telehealth or off-hours clinics) and (2) providing education about mental illness and mental health care to veterans, their families, health care providers, and others in their communities.[45]

Offering expanded options in mental health services aims to alleviate logistical challenges by making services available in more places at more times.[46] VHA policy requires that new patients requesting or referred for mental health services receive an initial assessment within 24 hours and a full evaluation appointment within 14 days; follow-up appointments for established patients must occur within 30 days.[47] The extent to which these policies are implemented in practice has been questioned in Congressional testimony, news media, and survey responses from both providers and patients.[48]

Educating veterans and others aims to increase understanding of mental health care and mental illness, reduce the associated stigma, and correct misconceptions about VHA care. For example, the VHA incorporates messages intended to reduce stigma into public health and outreach activities.

In addition, the VHA is working to integrate mental health and substance use evaluation and treatment services into other treatment settings, which both increases the convenience and reduces the stigma associated with seeking care.[49] Educational interventions are described in more detail in the next subsection.

Education

The VHA offers suicide prevention education to audiences within VHA facilities and in surrounding communities. VHA requires suicide prevention training for all VHA staff that interact with veterans, plus additional training for health care providers. In the community, the VHA provides education for veterans' families and community "guides."[50] Community guides are trained to recognize individuals who may be at risk of suicide and help them seek treatment. Evidence supports education of guides; however, they must be able to refer individuals to quality mental health services.[51] Thus, access to care and quality of care are essential.

Screening and Treatment

Some types of screening, pharmacotherapy, and psychotherapy are supported by evidence that they reduce the likelihood of suicide.[52]

VHA policy requires screening for a variety of risk factors, including depression, posttraumatic stress disorder (PTSD), problem drinking, traumatic brain injury (TBI), military sexual trauma (MST), and pain; veterans who screen positive must be offered follow-up evaluations and, if appropriate, treatment.[53]

An evaluation of VHA mental health care by the Altarum Institute and RAND Health finds that treatment in the VHA is generally better than in other systems on a variety of measures, but still has room for improvement.[54]

In particular, the evaluation finds that evidence-based treatments (both pharmacotherapy and psychotherapy), while widely available, are not usually provided.[55] Researchers based this finding on a review of medical records, which showed that prescriptions for medication were often not filled for as long as recommended and that psychotherapy, as documented, was often not delivered according to evidence-based guidelines.

Additionally, the evaluation found that assessment is lacking, both at the beginning of treatment and during treatment (to track progress).[56]

Even if a particular treatment is supported by evidence, it will not necessarily be effective for every patient.

The only way to know whether a patient is improving, holding steady, or growing worse is to assess his or her symptoms at intervals.

Limited Access to Lethal Means

The three most common means of completing suicide among the general population are firearms (50%), suffocation (24%), and poisoning (18%).[57] Evidence supports restricting access to lethal means (e.g., firearms, gas, drugs) as a way to reduce suicide rates.[58] The VHA has a gun safety program (as both a child safety initiative and a suicide prevention initiative), which includes distribution of gun safety literature and gun locks. The VHA also encourages demonstration projects and research on blister packaging medications as a way to reduce the incidence of medication overdoses.[59] Means restriction is a promising area still under investigation.[60]

Suicide Hotline

Suicide hotlines are telephone numbers individuals can call for help in crisis situations (e.g., at the moment they are considering suicide). Hotlines are generally toll-free and available around the clock. The Veterans Crisis Line is a joint effort of the VHA and SAMHSA.[61] The main line (1- 800-273-8255) is the National Suicide Prevention Lifeline, operated by SAMHSA.[62] Veterans (or others calling with concerns about veterans) may select option 1 to be directed to the VHA's Veterans Crisis Line, answered by staff at the COE in Canandaigua, New York. Callers may remain anonymous or disclose their identify in order to allow the COE staff to access their VA medical records during the call. Since the Veterans Crisis Line began in 2007, it has received over 500,000 calls, resulting in over 73,000 referrals to Suicide Prevention Coordinators for same-day or next-day service. The Veterans Crisis Line is supplemented by an online chat service (www.VeteransCrisisLine.net/chat) and support via text messaging (text 838255).[63]

The evidence base for suicide hotlines is not sufficient to determine their effectiveness in reducing suicide rates, due to the difficulties inherent in conducting such evaluations.[64] The confidentiality of suicide hotlines renders follow-up with each individual caller impossible. Moreover, national hotlines, such as those operated by SAMHSA and the VHA, serve a large geographic area. A range of other interventions may be in place in localities within the hotline's reach, such that any change in the suicide rate may not be attributable to the hotline.

Media Restrictions

Exposure to a suicide—whether through a personal relationship with the decedent or through media coverage—is a risk factor for suicide.[65] In this way, suicide sometimes seems to act as a contagion, resulting in suicide clusters as one suicide is followed by other imitative suicides. Following a completed suicide, news media may restrict how suicides are reported (e.g., not glamorizing suicide or not reporting the specific means), in an effort to reduce the likelihood of imitative suicides. Evidence has shown that this may reduce suicide at a particular site (e.g., a bridge); however, more evidence is needed to determine whether this approach reduces the overall rate of suicide.[66] The VA monitors depictions of suicide in the media and (working with other federal agencies and partners in academia) encourages both news and entertainment media to depict suicide in a manner that is ethical and responsible.[67]

Suicide Prevention Coordinators

Per department policy, every VA Medical Center has at least one suicide prevention coordinator, whose responsibilities include (among other things) tracking patients who have been identified as at high risk for suicide; the VHA's computerized patient record system enables clinicians to flag high-risk patients, and policy requires that safety plans be developed for them.[68] A safety plan is a written document, developed jointly by a patient and a clinician, that identifies strategies for coping in a crisis (e.g., recognizing warning signs and contacting family members, friends, or mental health providers). Outside the VA, the use of suicide prevention coordinators has not been widely adopted, although some components of the program (e.g., safety plans) are widely used. The suicide prevention coordinator program has been identified as a practice worth emulating by a DOD task force on suicide prevention.[69]

Potential Issues for Congress

A recurring theme in recommendations regarding VHA suicide prevention efforts is the need for the VHA to work in concert with other federal, state, and local government agencies; private for-profit and not-for-profit health care providers; veterans, their families, and their communities; and other individuals or organizations that might be able to help. Specific recommendations are organized in the following subsections, according to the public health framework for suicide prevention: surveillance, risk and protective factors, and interventions. Public laws addressing suicide prevention among veterans are described in the Appendix.

Potential Issues in Surveillance

As discussed earlier, three challenges in suicide surveillance are (1) timeliness of data, (2) accurate identification of decedents as veterans, and (3) consistent classification of deaths as suicides. Addressing these three challenges requires the involvement of entities other than VHA.

The Center for a New American Security (CNAS)[70] offers three recommendations related to the timeliness of data. First, CNAS recommends that "Congress should establish reasonable time requirements for states to provide death data to the CDC."[71] It should be noted that states, territories, and cities voluntarily share vital statistics with the CDC. Congress may be able to facilitate or motivate more rapid data sharing by providing resources or incentives.

Second, CNAS recommends ensuring that the CDC's ability to compile national death data expeditiously is not limited by a lack of resources.[72] Third, CNAS recommends that the annual analysis of veteran suicide data be coordinated among VA, DOD, and HHS.[73]

The VHA can identify decedents as veterans only if they are enrolled with the agency.[74] Identification of non-enrolled veterans relies on information gathered in the course of completing the death certificate or on supplemental information gathered as part of the National Violent Death Reporting System. VA researchers conducting a one-time study (not ongoing surveillance) combined information from the National Death Index with information from the DOD's Defense Manpower Data Center (DMDC) to identify suicides among veterans regardless of VA enrollment.[75] Congress may consider whether the DMDC is a source of information that can be used for suicide surveillance among veterans regardless of enrollment.

It is widely believed that inconsistent reporting of suicides across jurisdictions, as well as underreporting of suicides in general, limits the effectiveness of surveillance efforts.[76] Classification of a death as a suicide requires a determination that the death is both self-inflicted and intentional. Determining the decedent's intent is difficult, and coroners or medical examiners may feel pressure not to classify a death as suicide, due to the stigma associated with suicide.

Suicides may be underreported when the manner of death is misclassified as "undetermined" or "accidental" (e.g., poisonings or single-vehicle crashes). Additionally, each jurisdiction (state, territory, or city) has its own requirements for investigating deaths, leading to variability across jurisdictions. Congress may be able to facilitate or motivate more standardization by providing resources or incentives.

Potential Issues in Risk and Protective Factors

Recommendations in the area of risk and protective factors include collaboration and dialogue both among agencies involved in suicide prevention and across other areas of public health. CNAS suggests information sharing between the VA, DOD, and HHS[77] and recommends that the House and Senate Committees on Veterans' Affairs initiate discussions with the House and Senate Armed Services Committees to develop provisions addressing veteran suicide in the National Defense Authorization Act.[78] *Charting the Future* notes that suicide prevention tends to operate in its own silo, even though suicide has some of the same risk and protective factors as other public health problems. It recommends collaboration and dialogue between the suicide prevention effort and other public health efforts, stating, "Strong dialogue will help prevent the field from endlessly recreating wheels and spreading the limited funds too broadly to make a sustainable difference."[79]

Congress may choose to assess whether current levels of collaboration and dialogue are sufficient to ensure rapid dissemination of knowledge and avoid unnecessary duplication of effort. (Note that replication of studies is an integral part of the research process, so a distinction may be made between appropriate and unnecessary duplication of effort.) Congress may mandate, facilitate, or incentivize additional interagency coordination.

Potential Issues in Interventions

Three issues in VHA suicide prevention interventions that have come before Congress during hearings are (1) collaboration and dialogue, as discussed above; (2) an apparent gap between policy and practice; and (3) perceptions about mental illness and mental health care.[80]

If agencies (federal, state, or local) engage in ongoing collaboration and dialogue, sharing evaluations of existing interventions and research into new interventions, they may prevent unnecessary duplication of effort and help build the evidence base more quickly. The recommendations above regarding information sharing and collaboration pertain to intervention research as well.[81] *Charting the Future* advocates fast-tracking all phases of the intervention cycle (designing and pilot testing interventions, implementing interventions, and evaluating interventions), as well as the dissemination of the knowledge gained in each phase.[82] Moreover, congressional testimony has repeatedly called for increased use of non-VA resources, including other federal, state, and local government agencies; private for-profit and not-for-profit health care providers; veterans, their families, and their communities; and other individuals or organizations.[83] The use of non-VA resources might help suicide prevention interventions reach the majority of veterans who do not use VHA services.

A recurring theme in the area of suicide prevention interventions is the apparent gap between policy and practice. Examples of such a gap include the timeliness of mental health appointments and the use of evidence-based treatment. Increasing the timeliness of appointments may require congressional action in the form of additional resources in order to hire more providers, expand office space, or implement technologies such as telemedicine. Other gaps between policy and practice, such as the infrequent use of evidence-based treatment, may be possible for the VHA to address without additional resources; Congress may choose to continue exercising oversight in such areas.

Perceptions about mental illness and mental health care may affect whether veterans make use of treatment available to them. The belief that mental illness is a sign of weakness or something shameful may inhibit individuals or those around them from reaching out. Additionally, the belief that mental health care is not available, not appropriate, or not effective may discourage veterans from seeking care. Both stigma and mistaken beliefs may be reduced through discussions that address the facts of mental illness and mental health care. Thus congressional hearings on suicide, mental illness, or mental health care may have the unintended—but beneficial—consequence of reducing stigma and correcting misunderstandings about treatment.[84]

Appendix. Public Laws Addressing VA Suicide Prevention Efforts

Since Operations Enduring Freedom and Iraqi Freedom began, four public laws have addressed VHA suicide prevention efforts: the Joshua Omvig Veterans Suicide Prevention Act (P.L. 110- 110); the National Defense Authorization Act for Fiscal Year 2008 (P.L. 110-181); the Veterans' Benefits Improvement Act of 2008 (P.L. 110-389); and the Caregivers and Veterans Omnibus Health Services Act of 2010 (P.L. 111-163). Relevant provisions of each are summarized below.

Joshua Omvig Veterans Suicide Prevention Act

The Joshua Omvig Veterans Suicide Prevention Act (P.L. 110-110), enacted in 2007, required the VA Secretary to develop and implement a comprehensive suicide prevention program, and to report to Congress on the program.

The Congressional Budget Office estimated that implementing the Joshua Omvig Veterans Suicide Prevention Act would have "little, if any, cost," because the VA already had implemented or was planning to implement each of the specific requirements.[85]

The textbox below lists the required elements and additional authorized elements of the comprehensive suicide prevention program.

Joshua Omvig Veterans Suicide Prevention Act (P.L. 110-110)

Required elements of the comprehensive suicide prevention program include the following:

- mandatory suicide prevention training for appropriate VA staff and contractors;
- designation of a suicide prevention counselor at each VA medical center;
- outreach and education for veterans and their families to promote mental health;
- mental health assessments of veterans and referrals to appropriate treatment;
- availability of 24-hour mental health care for veterans;
- research on best practices for suicide prevention; and
- research on mental health among veterans with military sexual trauma.

Additional authorized (but not required) elements include the following:

- a 24-hour toll-free hotline staffed by trained mental health personnel;
- peer support counseling; and
- other actions to reduce the incidence of suicide among veterans.

National Defense Authorization Act for Fiscal Year 2008

Section 1611 of the National Defense Authorization Act for Fiscal Year 2008 (P.L. 110-181) directed the VA and DOD Secretaries to jointly develop a comprehensive care and transition policy for servicemembers recovering from serious injuries or illnesses related to their military service.

The law specified that the policy must address (among other things) the training and skills of health care professionals, recovery coordinators, and case managers, to ensure that they are able to detect and report early warning signs of suicidal thoughts or behaviors, along with other behavioral health concerns.

The law further specified that the policy must include tracking the notifications made by recovery care coordinators, medical care case managers, and nonmedical care managers to health care professionals regarding suicidal thoughts or behaviors, along with other behavioral health concerns.

A 2009 Government Accountability Office report indicates that DOD and VA have developed the relevant policies.[86]

Veterans' Benefits Improvement Act of 2008

Section 809 of the Veterans' Benefits Improvement Act of 2008 (P.L. 110-389) grants the VA Secretary authority to advertise in the media for various purposes, including suicide prevention.

Caregivers and Veterans Omnibus Health Services Act of 2010

Section 403 of the Caregivers and Veterans Omnibus Health Services Act of 2010 (P.L. 111-163) requires the VA Secretary to conduct a study to determine the number of veterans who died by suicide between January 1, 1999, and May 5, 2010 (i.e., the date of enactment). As of this writing, the study has not been completed.

End Notes

[1] See the *Appendix* for public laws addressing suicide among veterans.

[2] See, for example, U.S. Congress, Senate Committee on Veterans' Affairs, *VA Mental Health Care: Closing the Gaps*, 112th Cong., 1st sess., July 14, 2011; U.S. Congress, Senate Committee on Veterans' Affairs, *VA Mental Health Care: Addressing Wait Times and Access to Care*, 112th Cong., 1st sess., November 30, 2011; U.S. Congress, House Committee on Veterans' Affairs, Subcommittee on Health, *Understanding and Preventing Veteran Suicide*, 112th Cong., 1st sess., December 2, 2011.

[3] For suicide rates among veterans of Operations Enduring Freedom and Iraqi Freedom (OEF/OIF) using VA health care, and for a discussion of limitations of the data, see CRS Report R41921, *Suicide, PTSD, and Substance Use Among OEF/OIF Veterans Using VA Health Care: Facts and Figures*, by Erin Bagalman.

[4] This report focuses on the public health approach. A full discussion of the clinical approach to suicide prevention is beyond the scope of this report. The pharmacotherapy and psychotherapy mentioned in the "Screening and Treatment" section are examples of the clinical approach.

[5] U.S. Department of Health and Human Services (HHS), Public Health Service, *National Strategy for Suicide Prevention: Goals and Objectives for Action*, SMA01-3517, Rockville, MD, 2001, http://store.samhsa.gov/product/ SMA01-3517; hereinafter referred to as *National Strategy for Suicide Prevention*. The public health framework is described on pp. 29-40.

[6] Federal Working Group on Suicide Prevention, *National Strategy for Suicide Prevention: Compendium of Federal Activities*, 2009, http://www.samhsa.gov/mentalhealth/ NSSP Compendium_v2_March09.pdf. HHS agencies involved in suicide prevention include the Centers for Disease Control and Prevention (CDC), Indian Health Service (IHS), National Institute of Mental Health (NIMH), Substance Abuse and Mental Health Services Administration (SAMHSA), Health Resources and Services Administration (HRSA), Agency for Healthcare Research and Quality (AHRQ), and Administration on Aging (AoA).

[7] Veterans Health Administration, *VHA Strategic Plan for Suicide Prevention: FY 2009–2011*; hereinafter referred to as *VHA Strategic Plan*. The VHA Strategic Plan is based on both public health and clinical approaches; see Element 2.1.

[8] Suicide Prevention Resource Center and Suicide Prevention Action Network (SPAN), Charting the Future of Suicide Prevention: A 2010 Progress Review of the National Strategy and Recommendations for the Decade

Ahead, 2010, p. 18, http://www.sprc.org/library/ Charting TheFuture_Fullbook.pdf; hereinafter referred to as Charting the Future.

[9] *Charting the Future*, p. 11.

[10] See, for example, U.S. Congress, Senate Committee on Veterans' Affairs, *VA Mental Health Care: Closing the Gaps*, 112th Cong., 1st sess., July 14, 2011; U.S. Congress, Senate Committee on Veterans' Affairs, *VA Mental Health Care: Addressing Wait Times and Access to Care*, 112th Cong., 1st sess., November 30, 2011; U.S. Congress, House Committee on Veterans' Affairs, Subcommittee on Health, *Understanding and Preventing Veteran Suicide*, 112th Cong., 1st sess., December 2, 2011.

[11] Katherine E. Watkins and Harold Alan Pincus, *Veterans Health Administration Mental Health Program Evaluation: Capstone Report*, Altarum Institute and RAND Health, 2011, p. 153; hereinafter referred to as *VHA Mental Health Program Evaluation*.

[12] Suicide surveillance relies on information derived from death certificates. Both the legal authority for maintaining registries of deaths and the responsibility for issuing death certificates reside with individual states, territories, and two cities (Washington, DC, and New York, NY).

[13] The National Center for Health Statistics (NCHS) is part of the Centers for Disease Control and Prevention (CDC), within the Department of Health and Human Services (HHS). NCHS works cooperatively with state, territorial, and local jurisdictions to collect information from death certificates in the National Vital Statistics System (NVSS). NCHS extracts information from NVSS to create the National Death Index (NDI), a data set that can be combined with other data sets for research purposes. For more information, see CDC, National Center for Health Statistics, *About the National Death Index*, http://www.cdc.gov/nchs/data_access/ ndi/about_ndi.htm.

[14] VHA combines suicide data from the NDI with enrollment records to identify suicides among enrolled veterans. The enrollment file includes veterans receiving benefits from the Veterans Benefits Administration, even if the veterans are not receiving care from VHA.

[15] Researchers at the RAND Corporation summarized variation in suicide statistics across jurisdictions in four domains: (1) how suicides are defined or how ambiguous deaths are classified, (2) qualifications of professionals certifying a death as a suicide, (3) the extent to which possible suicide deaths are investigated, and (4) the quality of data management. Rajeev Ramchand et al., *The War Within: Preventing Suicide in the U.S. Military*, The RAND Corporation, 2011, p. 13, http://www.rand.org; hereinafter referred to as *The War Within*.

[16] The standard death certificate allows officials to indicate if a decedent has ever served in the U.S. Armed Forces; however, this indication captures both veterans and current servicemembers, with no means of distinguishing between the two. Also, the individual responsible for completing the death certificate may not know whether the decedent is a veteran.

[17] See textbox in the Introduction.

[18] *VHA Strategic Plan*, Element 7.1.

[19] HHS, CDC, *Fiscal Year 2012 Justification of Estimates for Appropriation Committees*.

[20] HHS, CDC, *National Violent Death Reporting System*, http://www.cdc.gov/violenc eprevention/nvdrs and http://www.cdc.gov/ncipc/wisqars/NVDRS.

[21] HHS, CDC, *Fiscal Year 2012 Justification of Estimates for Appropriation Committees*.

[22] HHS, CDC, National Center for Injury Prevention and Control, Division of Violence Prevention, *Preventing Suicide: Program Activities Guide*, Atlanta, GA, 2010, http://www. cdc.gov/ViolencePrevention/pub /PreventingSuicide.html.

[23] Ibid.

[24] *Charting the Future*, p. 30.

[25] Centers for Disease Control and Prevention, *Suicide: Risk and Protective Factors*, Atlanta, GA, http://www.cdc. gov/ViolencePrevention/suicide/riskprotectivefactors.html.

[26] HHS, National Institutes of Health (NIH), National Institute of Mental Health, *Publications about Suicide Prevention*, http://www.nimh.nih.gov/health/publications/suicide-prevention-listing.shtml; and National Institute of Mental Health, *Science News about Suicide Prevention*, http://www.nimh.nih.gov/science-news/science-news-aboutsuicide-prevention. shtml.

[27] SAMHSA asks about these topics in the National Survey on Drug Use and Health (NSDUH). See HHS, CDC, *Morbidity and Mortality Weekly Report: Suicidal Thoughts and Behaviors Among Adults ≥ 18 Years—United States, 2008 – 2009*, October 21, 2011, http://www.cdc. gov/mmwr/preview/mmwrhtml/ss6013a1.htm.

[28] HHS, CDC, *Suicide: Facts at a Glance*, 2009, http://www.cdc.gov/violenceprevention /pdf/ suicide-datasheet-a.pdf.

[29] For example, although the single strongest predictor of a completed suicide is a prior suicide attempt, most people who attempt suicide do not subsequently complete suicide, and most people who complete suicides have no history of prior attempts. See *The War Within* and Joel Paris, "Predicting and Preventing Suicide: Do We Know Enough to Do Either?," *Harvard Review of Psychiatry*, vol. 14, no. 5 (2006), pp. 233-240.

[30] The ORD supports research through four research divisions: Biomedical Laboratory Research and Development (BLR&D), Clinical Science Research and Development (CSR&D), Rehabilitation Research and Development (RR&D), and Health Services Research and Development (HSR&D).

[31] A search for "suicide*" at http://www.hsrd.research.va.gov/research/ yields dozens of suicide-related studies conducted within ORD's Health Services Research and Development (HSR&D) Service; some of the resulting studies investigate risk factors and/or protective factors.

[32] VA, VHA, Health Services Research and Development, *Suicide Among Veterans: Using the VA Depression Registry to Inform Care*, Study IIR 04-211, http://www.hsrd.research.va. gov/research/abstracts.cfm?Project_ID=2141695453.

[33] VA, VHA, Health Services Research and Development, *Suicidality: Correlates and Impact on Preference-Weighted Health Status of Veterans in VA Primary Care*, Study SHP 08-160, http://www.hsrd.research.va. gov/research/ abstracts.cfm?Project_ID=2141698711.

[34] U.S. Congress, Committee of Conference, *Making Appropriations for Military Quality of Life Functions of the Department of Defense, Military Construction, the Department of Veterans Affairs, and Related Agencies for the Fiscal Year Ending September 30, 2006, and for Other Purposes*, report to accompany H.R. 2528, 109th Cong., 1st sess., November 18, 2005, H.Rept. 109-305 (Washington: GPO, 2006), p. 39. The committee report directed the VHA "to place more emphasis on psychiatric care of our veterans by designating three centers of excellence to focus on mental health/PTSD needs. These three centers will be established at Waco Medical Center, Texas; San Diego Medical Center, California; and the Canandaigua Medical Center, New York."

[35] VA, VHA, VISN 2 Center of Excellence at Canandaigua, http://www.mirecc.va.gov/ docs/ 2010InfoSheets/ VISN_2_CoE_Canandaigua_Info_Sheet_2010.pdf.

[36] P.L. 104-262, Veterans' Health Care Eligibility Reform Act of 1996, enacted 10/09/1996 (38 U.S.C. § 7320).

[37] VA, VHA, *MIRECC of the VA Rocky Mountain Network (VISN 19 MIRECC)*, http://www. mirecc.va.gov/visn19/ index.asp.

[38] VA, VHA, VISN 19 MIRECC, *Examining Prolonged Grief Disorder and Its Relationship to Self-Directed Violence (SDV) Among Veterans*, http://www.mirecc.va.gov/visn19/ studies/ grief/index.asp.

[39] VA, VHA, VISN 19 MIRECC, *Neurobiology Of Suicide Risk In Traumatic Brain Injury And Substance Abuse*, http://www.mirecc.va.gov/visn19/studies/tbi_sud/index.asp.

[40] One goal of the Mental Health Quality Enhancement Research Initiative (QUERI) within ORD is to "[d]evelop and implement evidence-based suicide prevention strategies." See VA Mental Health QUERI Center, *Strategic Plan*, November 2008, http://www.queri.research. va.gov/about/strategic_plans/mh.pdf#page=21; and VA Mental Health QUERI Center, *Fact Sheet*, June 2011, http://www.queri.research.va.gov /about/ factsheets/mh_ factsheet.pdf.

[41] The COE at Canandaigua evaluates implementation of suicide prevention initiatives.

[42] For example, the MIRECC of the VA Rocky Mountain Network is conducting a pilot program to determine whether providing prescription medication in blister packages (rather than bottles) reduces the likelihood of overdose. Veterans Health Administration, Blister Packaging Medication to Increase Treatment Adherence and Clinical Response: Impact on Suicide-Related Morbidity and Mortality, http://www.mirecc.va.gov/ projects/blisterpack /index.asp.

[43] *The War Within*, p. 13.

[44] Ibid.

[45] U.S. Government Accountability Office, *VA Mental Health: Number of Veterans Receiving Care, Barriers Faced, and Efforts to Increase Access*, GAO-12-12, October 14, 2011, pp. 15-17, http://www.gao .gov/products/GAO-12-12.

[46] Ibid. Examples of expanded options include increasing use of telemental health services and call centers (i.e., telephone counseling), integrating mental health services into primary care settings, increasing the number of mental health staff and mental health clinic hours, and adding more Vet Centers.

[47] VA, VHA, *Uniform Mental Health Services in VA Medical Centers and Clinics*, VHA Handbook 1160.01, September 11, 2008.

[48] U.S. Congress, Senate Committee on Veterans' Affairs, *VA Mental Health Care: Closing the Gaps*, 112th Cong., 1st sess., July 14, 2011; U.S. Congress, Senate Committee on Veterans' Affairs, *VA Mental Health Care: Addressing Wait Times and Access to Care*, 112th Cong., 1st sess., November 30, 2011; Gregg Zoroya and Paul

Monies, "Lag in Mental Health Care Found at a Third of VA Hospitals," *USA Today*, November 9, 2011, http://www. usatoday.com/news/ military/story/2011-11-09/veterans-mental-health-care/ 51143216/1; and *VHA Mental Health Program Evaluation*.

[49] *VHA Strategic Plan*, Elements 4.1, 4.2, and 4.3.

[50] *VHA Strategic Plan*, Element 9.1, 9.2, 9.3, and 9.4.

[51] *The War Within*. Outside the VHA, the term "gatekeeper" (rather than "guide") is generally used.

[52] *The War Within*.

[53] *VHA Strategic Plan*, Element 6.2.

[54] *VHA Mental Health Program Evaluation*, p. 153.

[55] *VHA Mental Health Program Evaluation*. For example, among veterans for whom maintenance medication is recommended, less than one-third received the recommended continuous treatment (p. 160). Similarly, among veterans receiving psychotherapy, "most did not include elements of an evidence-based modality" (p. 154).

[56] *VHA Mental Health Program Evaluation*. Less than two-thirds of veterans in a new treatment episode "have a documented assessment of their housing and employment needs" (p. 161). Among veterans with major depressive disorder who were receiving psychotherapy, less than a quarter (23%) "had documentation of an assessment of response to psychotherapy" (p. 155).

[57] Mechanism of injury for suicides among the general U.S. population in CY2007 identified from Centers for Disease Control and Prevention, National Center for Health Statistics. *Compressed Mortality File 1999-2007. CDC WONDER On-line Database, compiled from Compressed Mortality File 1999-2007 Series 20 No. 2M, 2010*, http://wonder.cdc.gov/cmf-icd10.html.

[58] J. John Mann et al., "Suicide Prevention Strategies: A Systematic Review," *Journal of the American Medical Association*, vol. 294, no. 16 (October 26, 2005), pp. 2064-2074.

[59] VHA Strategic Plan, Elements 10.4 and 10.6; and VA, Blister Packaging Medication to Increase Treatment Adherence and Clinical Response: Impact on Suicide-Related Morbidity and Mortality, http://www. mirecc. va.gov/ projects/blisterpack/index.asp.

[60] J. John Mann et al., "Suicide Prevention Strategies: A Systematic Review," *Journal of the American Medical Association*, vol. 294, no. 16 (October 26, 2005), pp. 2064-2074.

[61] *VHA Strategic Plan*, Element 6.10.

[62] Substance Abuse and Mental Health Services Administration, *National Suicide Prevention Lifeline*, http://www.suicidepreventionlifeline.org/.

[63] U.S. Congress, House Committee on Veterans' Affairs, Subcommittee on Health, *Understanding and Preventing Veteran Suicide*, 112th Cong., 1st sess., December 2, 2011, testimony of Jan E. Kemp, RN, Ph.D., National Mental Health Director for Suicide Prevention, Veterans Heath Administration, U.S. Department of Veterans Affairs.

[64] J. John Mann et al., "Suicide Prevention Strategies: A Systematic Review," *Journal of the American Medical Association*, vol. 294, no. 16 (October 26, 2005), pp. 2064-2074.

[65] *National Strategy for Suicide Prevention*, p. 36.

[66] J. John Mann et al., "Suicide Prevention Strategies: A Systematic Review," *Journal of the American Medical Association*, vol. 294, no. 16 (October 26, 2005), pp. 2064-2074.

[67] *VHA Strategic Plan*, Elements 11.1 and 11.2.

[68] VA, Office of Inspector General, *Healthcare Inspection: Evaluation of Suicide Prevention Program Implementation in VHA Facilities, January–June 2009*, Report No. 09-00326-223, Washington, DC, September 22, 2009, http://www.va.gov/oig/54/reports/VAOIG-09-00326-223.pdf; and VA, Office of Inspector General, *Combined Assessment Program Summary Report: Re-Evaluation of Suicide Safety Plan Practices in Veterans Health Administration Facilities*, Report No. 11-01380-128, Washington, DC, March 22, 2011, http://www.va.gov/oig/CAP/ VAOIG-11-01380-128.pdf.

[69] Department of Defense Task Force on the Prevention of Suicide by Members of the Armed Forces, *The Challenge and the Promise: Strengthening the Force, Preventing Suicide, and Saving Lives*, August 2010, pp. 55, 89, http://www.health.mil/dhb/subcommittees-tfpsmaf.cfm; hereinafter referred to as *The Challenge and the Promise*.

[70] CNAS is a 501(c)3 tax-exempt nonprofit organization located in Washington; it describes itself as independent and non-partisan. (http://www.cnas.org/about).

[71] Margaret Harrell and Nancy Berglass, *Losing the Battle: The Challenge of Military Suicide*, Center for a New American Security, Washington, DC, October 2011, p. 9; hereinafter referred to as *Losing the Battle*.

[72] Ibid.

[73] Ibid.

[74] The enrollment file includes veterans receiving benefits from the Veterans Benefits Administration, even if the veterans are not receiving care from VHA.

[75] Han K. Kang and Tim A. Bullman, "Letter: Risk of Suicide Among US Veterans After Returning From the Iraq or Afghanistan War Zones," *Journal of the American Medical Association*, vol. 300, no. 6 (2008), pp. 652-653. The study was limited to veterans who served in Operations Enduring Freedom and/or Iraqi Freedom and who were separated alive from active duty between October 2001 and December 2005.

[76] See for example Stefan Timmermans, "Suicide determination and the professional authority of medical examiners.," *American Sociological Review*, vol. 70, no. 2 (2005), pp. 311-333; Hugh P. Whitt, "Where did the bodies go? The social construction of suicide data, New York City, 1976-1992," *Sociological Inquiry*, vol. 76, no. 2 (2006), pp. 166- 187; M.J. Breiding and B. Wiersema, "Variability of undetermined manner of death classification in the U.S.," *Injury Prevention*, vol. 12(Suppl II) (2006), pp. ii49-ii54.

[77] *Losing the Battle*, p. 9.

[78] Ibid.

[79] *Charting the Future*, p. 40.

[80] U.S. Congress, Senate Committee on Veterans' Affairs, *VA Mental Health Care: Closing the Gaps*, 112th Cong., 1st sess., July 14, 2011; U.S. Congress, Senate Committee on Veterans' Affairs, *VA Mental Health Care: Addressing Wait Times and Access to Care*, 112th Cong., 1st sess., November 30, 2011; U.S. Congress, House Committee on Veterans' Affairs, Subcommittee on Health, *Understanding and Preventing Veteran Suicide*, 112th Cong., 1st sess., December 2, 2011.

[81] *Losing the Battle*, p. 9; and *Charting the Future*, p. 40.

[82] *Charting the Future*, p. 40.

[83] U.S. Congress, Senate Committee on Veterans' Affairs, *VA Mental Health Care: Addressing Wait Times and Access to Care*, 112th Cong., 1st sess., November 30, 2011; U.S. Congress, House Committee on Veterans' Affairs, Subcommittee on Health, *Understanding and Preventing Veteran Suicide*, 112th Cong., 1st sess., December 2, 2011.

[84] U.S. Congress, Senate Committee on Veterans' Affairs, *VA Mental Health Care: Closing the Gaps*, 112th Cong., 1st sess., July 14, 2011. Senator Murray mentioned stigma in her opening statement, and it was discussed at several points.

[85] U.S. Congressional Budget Office, *Cost Estimate for H.R. 327 Joshua Omvig Veterans Suicide Prevention Act*, March 19, 2007; and U.S. Congressional Budget Office, *Cost Estimate for S.4797 Joshua Omvig Veterans Suicide Prevention Act*, July 10, 2007.

[86] U.S. Government Accountability Office, *Recovering Servicemembers: DOD and VA Have Jointly Developed the Majority of Required Policies but Challenges Remain*, GAO-09-728, July 2009, p. 25.

In: Veteran Injuries, Disorders and Medical Care Service
Editors: Jessica Michaels and Jesse E. Levine
ISBN: 978-1-62081-302-7

Chapter 6

VA MENTAL HEALTH: NUMBER OF VETERANS RECEIVING CARE, BARRIERS FACED, AND EFFORTS TO INCREASE ACCESS*

United States Government Accountability Office

WHY GAO DID THIS STUDY

In fiscal year 2010, the Department of Veterans Affairs (VA) provided health care to about 5.2 million veterans. Recent legislation has increased many Operations Enduring Freedom (OEF) and Iraqi Freedom (OIF) veterans' priority for accessing VA's health care, and concerns have been raised about the extent to which VA is providing mental health care to eligible veterans of all eras. There also are concerns that barriers may hinder some veterans from accessing needed mental health care.

GAO was asked to provide information on veterans who receive mental health care from VA. In this report, GAO provides information on (1) how many veterans received mental health care from VA from fiscal years 2006 through 2010, (2) key barriers that may hinder veterans from accessing mental health care from VA, and (3) VA efforts to increase veterans' access to VA mental health care. GAO obtained data from VA's Northeast Program Evaluation Center (NEPEC) on the number of veterans who received mental health care from VA. The number of veterans represents a unique count of veterans; veterans were counted only once, even if they received care multiple times during a fiscal year or across the 5-year period. GAO also reviewed literature published from 2006 to 2011, reviewed VA documents, and interviewed officials from VA and veterans service organizations (VSO).

* This is an edited, reformatted and augmented version of the Highlights of GAO-12-12, a report to the Ranking Member, Committee on Veterans' Affairs, House of Representatives, dated October 2011.

WHAT GAO FOUND

Over the 5-year period from fiscal years 2006 through 2010, about 2.1 million unique veterans received mental health care from VA. (See figure.) Each year the number of veterans receiving mental health care increased, from about 900,000 in fiscal year 2006 to about 1.2 million in fiscal year 2010. OEF/OIF veterans accounted for an increasing proportion of veterans receiving care during this period.

The key barriers identified from the literature that may hinder veterans from accessing mental health care from VA, which were corroborated through interviews, are stigma, lack of understanding or awareness of mental health care, logistical challenges to accessing mental health care, and concerns about VA's care, such as concerns that VA's services are primarily for older veterans. Many of these barriers are not necessarily unique to veterans accessing mental health care from VA, but may affect anyone accessing mental health care from any provider. Veterans may be affected by barriers differently based on demographic factors, such as age and gender. For example, younger OEF/OIF veterans and female veterans may perceive that VA's services are primarily for someone else, such as older veterans or male veterans.

VA has implemented several efforts to increase veterans' access to mental health care, including integrating mental health care into primary care. VA also has implemented efforts to educate veterans, their families, health care providers, and other community stakeholders about mental health conditions and VA's mental health care. According to VA officials, these efforts help get veterans into care by reducing, and in some cases eliminating, the barriers that may hinder them from accessing care.

GAO provided a draft of this report to VA for comment. In its response, VA provided technical comments, which were incorporated as appropriate.

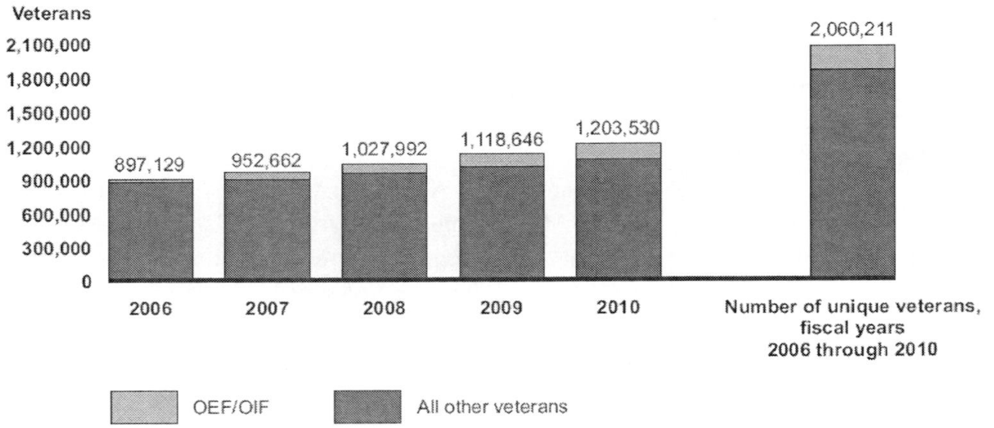

Source: GAO analysis of NEPEC data.

Number of Veterans Who Received Mental Health Care from VA, Fiscal Years 2006 through 2010

ABBREVIATIONS

NEPEC	Northeast Program Evaluation Center
OEF	Operation Enduring Freedom
OIF	Operation Iraqi Freedom
PTSD	post-traumatic stress disorder
VA	Department of Veterans Affairs
VHA	Veterans Health Administration
VSO	veterans service organization

October 14, 2011

The Honorable Bob Filner
Ranking Member
Committee on Veterans' Affairs
House of Representatives

Dear Mr. Filner:

In fiscal year 2010, the Department of Veterans Affairs (VA), which operates one of the largest health care delivery systems in the nation, provided health care to about 5.2 million veterans. VA provides care to eligible veterans from all eras of service,[1] including World War II, Korea, Vietnam, Gulf War, and most recently, military operations in Afghanistan and Iraq—Operation Enduring Freedom (OEF) and Operation Iraqi Freedom (OIF), respectively.[2] Recent legislation has increased many OEF/OIF veterans' priority for accessing VA's health care.[3]

Given the increased focus on OEF/OIF veterans, concerns have been raised by some, including veterans service organizations (VSO), about the extent to which VA is providing mental health care to eligible veterans of all eras. We have previously reported that VA has experienced an increased demand for its mental health care—including care for conditions such as post-traumatic stress disorder (PTSD), depression, and substance abuse.[4] Additionally, there are concerns that barriers— such as distance from a VA treatment facility or stigma associated with mental health care—may hinder some veterans from accessing needed mental health care. When veterans do not receive the mental health care they need, wide-ranging and negative implications for their physical, work, family, and social functioning can result. For example, mental health conditions can lead to increased risks of unemployment, homelessness, and suicide.

You expressed interest in obtaining information on veterans who receive mental health care from VA. In this report, we provide information on (1) how many veterans received mental health care from VA from fiscal years 2006 through 2010, (2) key barriers that may hinder veterans from accessing mental health care from VA, and (3) efforts VA has implemented to increase veterans' access to VA mental health care.

To perform our work, we obtained data from VA's Northeast Program Evaluation Center (NEPEC)[5] on the number of veterans who received mental health care from VA from fiscal years 2006 through 2010. For the purposes of this report, we defined mental health care as the care provided to veterans with mental health conditions. A veteran was counted as having a mental health condition if, at any point in the fiscal year, his or her medical record indicated at least two outpatient encounters with any mental health diagnosis (with at least one encounter having a primary mental health diagnosis) or an inpatient stay in which the veteran had any mental health diagnosis.[6] Additionally, the number of veterans represents a unique count of veterans; veterans were counted only once, even if they received care multiple times during a fiscal year or across the 5-year period. To assess the reliability of the data NEPEC provided us, we discussed with NEPEC officials their methodology and data collection techniques for obtaining and using the data, the data checks that NEPEC performed, as well as any limitations officials identified in the data. In addition, we did our own review of NEPEC's programming and methodological approaches using data file documentation, code book and file dictionaries, and programming logs NEPEC officials provided. We determined that the data were sufficiently reliable for our purposes.

To identify the key barriers that may hinder veterans from accessing mental health care from VA, we searched research databases, such as MEDLINE and PsycINFO, that included peer-reviewed journals to capture relevant literature published on or between January 1, 2006, and March 3, 2011. We also reviewed relevant literature that was cited in articles from our original search or recommended to us during the course of our research. To corroborate the barriers we identified in the literature, we interviewed officials from (1) several VA offices—the Office of Mental Health Services, the Office of Mental Health Operations, the Office of Rural Health, the Office of Research and Development, and Readjustment Counseling Services; (2) several mental health–focused VA research centers—the Mental Illness Research, Education and Clinical Center, the Serious Mental Illness Treatment Resource and Evaluation Center, the Center for Chronic Disease Outcomes Research, and the National Center for PTSD; (3) several VA mental health and primary care providers;[7] and (4) a judgmental sample of VSOs.[8] We defined "key barriers" as those that the majority of VA and VSO officials we interviewed said could have the greatest impact on veterans. As a result, we do not report an exhaustive list of all potential barriers that veterans may face.

Finally, to identify the efforts VA has implemented to increase veterans' access to VA mental health care, we reviewed documentation and interviewed officials from the same VA offices and mental health–focused VA research centers that we interviewed to corroborate the barriers for veterans. We compiled a list of efforts based on those that had been implemented and were national in scope. As a result, we do not report an exhaustive list of all VA efforts. In addition, we did not assess the extent to which VA has fully implemented these efforts or their effectiveness, including the extent to which the efforts eliminate or diminish barriers that may hinder veterans from accessing mental health care.

We conducted our work from November 2010 to October 2011 in accordance with all sections of GAO's Quality Assurance Framework that are relevant to our objectives. The framework requires that we plan and perform the engagement to obtain sufficient and appropriate evidence to meet our stated objectives and to discuss any limitations in our work. We believe that the information and data obtained, and the analysis conducted, provide a reasonable basis for any findings and conclusions. See appendix I for a complete description of our scope and methodology.

BACKGROUND

VA manages access to services in relation to available resources through a priority system established by law.[9] The order of priorities is generally based on service-connected disability, income, or other special status, such as having been a prisoner of war.[10] Additionally, Congress has stipulated that certain combat veterans discharged from active duty on or after January 2003 are eligible for priority enrollment.

VA Mental Health Care

VA provides mental health care—for conditions such as PTSD, depression, and substance abuse disorders—in a variety of facilities, including medical centers, community-based outpatient clinics, and rehabilitation treatment programs. These facilities may include both specialty mental health care settings and other settings. Specialty mental health settings, including mental health clinics, primarily provide mental health services. Other settings may provide mental health services but focus primarily on other types of care, such as primary care.

VA also provides counseling services that focus on mental health issues through its Vet Centers, a nationwide system of community-based centers that VA established separately from other facilities. The counseling services provided by Vet Centers differ from the mental health services provided by other VA facilities in that they focus on counseling to assist combat veterans in readjusting from wartime military service to civilian life but do not diagnose veterans' mental health conditions. Veterans needing more acute care—for example, veterans with multiple mental health conditions, such as severe PTSD and depression, or those who pose a risk of harm to themselves or others—are often referred to VA medical centers for diagnosis and treatment.

Veteran Eras of Military Service

VA groups veterans by dates—or era—of their military service based on provisions in federal law.[11] (See table 1.)

VA estimates that as of September 30, 2011, there were approximately 22.2 million living veterans. OEF/OIF veterans represented approximately 12 percent (2.6 million) of that total.

MORE THAN 2 MILLION UNIQUE VETERANS RECEIVED MENTAL HEALTH CARE FROM VA OVER THE 5-YEAR PERIOD FROM FISCAL YEARS 2006 THROUGH 2010

Over the 5-year period from fiscal years 2006 through 2010, about 2.1 million unique veterans received mental health care from VA.[12] Each year the number of veterans receiving care increased—from about 900,000 in fiscal year 2006 to about 1.2 million in fiscal year

2010. (See figure 1.) VA provided this mental health care to veterans in both specialty mental health care and other settings, such as primary care clinics staffed with mental health providers.[13] (See app. II for information on the number of veterans receiving mental health care in specialty mental health care and other settings.)

Although the number of veterans receiving mental health care from VA increased for both OEF/OIF veterans and veterans of other eras of service, as shown in figure 1, OEF/OIF veterans accounted for an increasing proportion of the veterans receiving care. Specifically, the proportion of OEF/OIF veterans receiving mental health care from VA out of the total number of veterans receiving mental health care increased from 4 percent in fiscal year 2006 to 12 percent in fiscal year 2010. Nonetheless, veterans from earlier eras, such as Vietnam, accounted for approximately 90 percent of the 2.1 million veterans receiving care at VA over the 5-year period from fiscal years 2006 through 2010, although the proportion decreased from 96 percent in fiscal year 2006 to 88 percent in fiscal year 2010. VA officials indicated that the increasing proportion of OEF/OIF veterans receiving mental health care is not unexpected because of the nature of OEF/OIF veterans' military service—veterans of this era typically had intense and frequent deployments. In addition, according to VA officials, VA has made changes in its mental health screening protocols that may have resulted in more mental health conditions being diagnosed among veterans entering the VA system. For example, VA requires veterans treated in primary care settings to be screened for mental health conditions such as PTSD, depression, substance abuse disorders, as well as a history of military sexual trauma.

Table 1. Veteran Eras of Military Service

Era of military service	Years	Estimated number of living veterans, as of September 30, 2011[a]
World War II	Dec. 7, 1941 – Dec. 31, 1946	1.7 million
Korea	June 27, 1950 – Jan. 31, 1955	2.3 million
Vietnam	Feb. 28, 1961 – May 7, 1975	7.4 million
Persian Gulf War[b]	Aug. 2, 1990 – present	3.3 million
OEF/OIF[b]	October 2001 – present	2.6 million
Peacetime	Any dates outside of specified eras of service	5.7 million

Source: GAO analysis of 38 U.S.C. § 101 and VA VetPop2007 data.

[a] Estimates are from VetPop2007, a VA model for estimating the number of living veterans using U.S. Census Bureau and Department of Defense data. There were an estimated 22.2 million total living veterans as of September 30, 2011. This total is less than the sum of the number of living veterans from the individual eras of military service because some veterans served in multiple eras.

[b] OEF/OIF is a set of military operations that is considered part of the Persian Gulf War. Although most veterans who have served since 2001 served in OEF/OIF, there are some veterans who served in the Persian Gulf War after 2001 who did not serve in OEF/OIF. For the purposes of this report, we consider OEF/OIF to be an era of military service, and we use the time frame corresponding to the beginning of OEF, the operation with the earliest start date. In addition, we include veterans of Operation New Dawn—the name given to combat in Afghanistan after September 2010—in the OEF/OIF era of military service. Finally, for the estimated number of living veterans, veterans who served in both the Persian Gulf War era and the OEF/OIF era are counted in the OEF/OIF era.

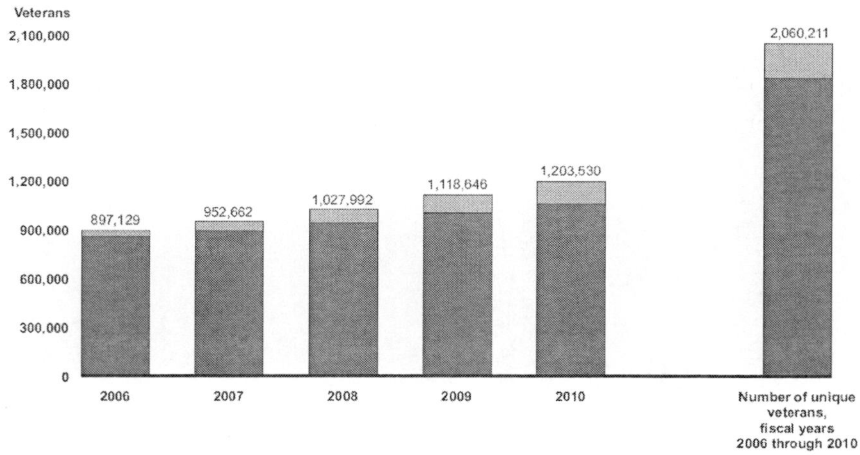

	2006	2007	2008	2009	2010	Number of unique veterans, fiscal years 2006 through 2010
OEF/OIF	34,559 (4%)	55,343 (6%)	83,947 (8%)	113,277 (10%)	139,167 (12%)	213,781 (10%)
All other veterans	862,570 (96%)	897,319 (94%)	944,045 (92%)	1,005,369 (90%)	1,064,363 (88%)	1,846,430 (90%)

Source: GAO analysis of NEPEC data.

Notes: The number of veterans represents a unique count of veterans; veterans were counted only once, even if they received care multiple times during a fiscal year or across the 5-year period.

We defined mental health care as the care provided to veterans with mental health conditions. A veteran was counted as having a mental health condition if, at any point in the fiscal year, his or her medical record indicated at least two outpatient encounters with any mental health diagnosis (with at least one encounter having a primary mental health diagnosis) or an inpatient stay in which the veteran had any mental health diagnosis.

Figure 1. Number of Veterans Who Received Mental Health Care from VA, Fiscal Years 2006 through 2010.

Additionally, the 2.1 million veterans receiving mental health care from VA accounted for almost a third of the 7.2 million total unique veterans receiving any type of health care from VA over the 5-year period from fiscal years 2006 through 2010.[14] Specifically, 38 percent of all OEF/OIF veterans and 28 percent of all other veterans receiving any health care during this time period received mental health care. (See figure 2.)

The five most common diagnostic categories for veterans receiving mental health care from VA in fiscal year 2010 were adjustment reaction, depressive disorder, episodic mood disorder, neurotic disorder, and substance abuse disorder. (See table 2.) Within each diagnostic category, there are specific mental health diagnoses; for example, PTSD is one of the diagnoses within the adjustment reaction category. Although veterans of all eras had similar diagnoses, the likelihood of experiencing diagnoses in any one category varied by era. Specifically, almost twice as many OEF/OIF veterans had diagnoses within the adjustment reaction category compared to the next most common diagnostic category—depressive disorder. In comparison, for veterans of all other eras, depressive disorder was the most common diagnostic category, but it was closely followed by adjustment reaction. According to VA officials, the higher relative incidence of adjustment reaction (including PTSD) among OEF/OIF veterans may be due to many factors, including the length and frequency of their deployments and a better understanding of how to identify and diagnose PTSD among mental health care providers.

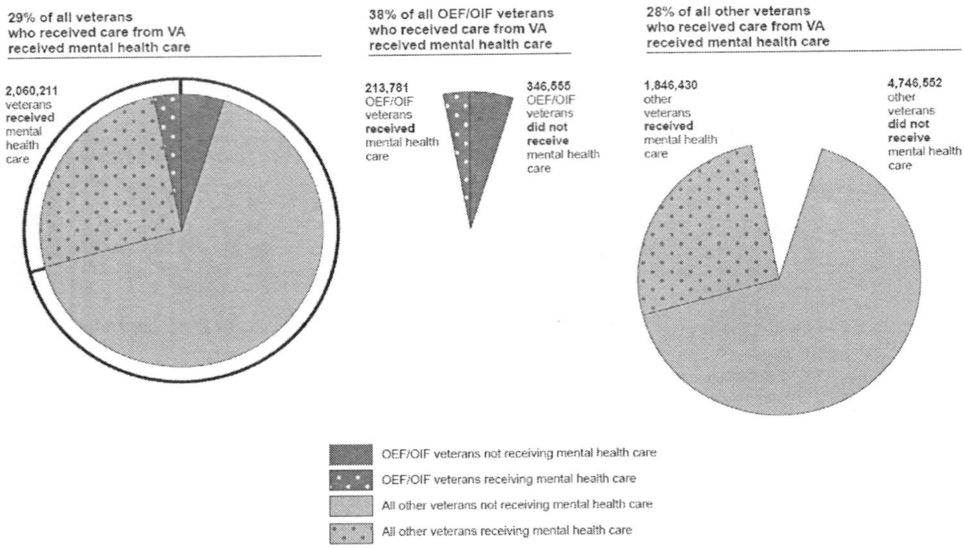

Source: GAO analysis of NEPEC data.

Notes: The number of veterans represents a unique count of veterans; veterans were counted only once, even if they received care multiple times across the 5-year period.

We defined mental health care as the care provided to veterans with mental health conditions. A veteran was counted as having a mental health condition if, at any point in the fiscal year, his or her medical record indicated at least two outpatient encounters with any mental health diagnosis (with at least one encounter having a primary mental health diagnosis) or an inpatient stay in which the veteran had any mental health diagnosis.

Figure 2. Percentage of Veterans Receiving Mental Health Care from VA as a Percentage of the Total Number of Veterans Receiving Any Health Care from VA over the 5-Year Period from Fiscal Years 2006 through 2010.

Stigma, Lack of Understanding of Mental Health, Logistical Challenges, and Concerns about VA May Hinder Veterans from Accessing Care

The key barriers we identified from the literature that may hinder veterans from accessing mental health care from VA, which were corroborated through interviews with VA and VSO officials, are stigma, lack of understanding or awareness of mental health care, logistical challenges to accessing mental health care, and concerns about VA's care. (See table 3 for a description of each of these key barriers.) For example, stigma—negative personal or societal beliefs about mental health conditions or mental health care—may discourage veterans from accessing care. According to VA and VSO officials we spoke with, some veterans may have concerns that if colleagues or employers find out they are receiving mental health care, their careers will be negatively affected.

Table 2. Five Most Common Diagnostic Categories for Veterans Receiving Mental Health Care from VA, Fiscal Year 2010

Diagnostic category[a]	Description	Number of OEF/OIF veterans	Number of all other veterans	Total number of veterans
Adjustment reaction	A group of mental health diagnoses, including PTSD, characterized by an emotional and behavioral reaction that develops within 3 months of a life stress, and which is stronger or greater than what would be expected for the type of event that occurred.	109,850 (includes 96,916 with PTSD diagnosis)	465,448 (includes 383,832 with PTSD diagnosis)	575,298 (includes 480,748 with PTSD diagnosis)
Depressive disorder	A group of mental health diagnoses that reflect a sad or irritable mood exceeding normal sadness or grief.	57,639	477,029	534,668
Episodic mood disorder	A group of mental health diagnoses best recognized by depression or mania that can have potentially severe health consequences.	38,715	352,651	391,366
Neurotic disorder	A group of mental health diagnoses characterized by symptoms such as phobias, obsessive thoughts, and compulsive actions, or by losses of specific bodily functions.	45,252	343,562	388,814
Substance abuse disorder	A group of mental health diagnoses arising from the abuse of alcohol or drugs.	36,797	326,417	363,214

Source: GAO analysis of NEPEC data.

Notes: Veterans could have more than one diagnosis; therefore the numbers do not add to the 1.2 million veterans receiving mental health care from VA in fiscal year 2010.

We defined mental health care as the care provided to veterans with mental health conditions. A veteran was counted as having a mental health condition if, at any point in the fiscal year, his or her medical record indicated at least two outpatient encounters with any mental health diagnosis (with at least one encounter having a primary mental health diagnosis) or an inpatient stay in which the veteran had any mental health diagnosis.

[a] Diagnostic categories are based on International Classification of Diseases, Ninth Revision, codes.

Many of these barriers are not necessarily unique to veterans accessing mental health care from VA, but may affect anyone accessing mental health care from any provider. According to the Substance Abuse and Mental Health Services Administration's 2008 National Survey on Drug Use and Health, approximately 5 million adults who reported an unmet need for mental health care reported similar barriers.[15] In particular, survey participants cited the following as barriers: a belief that the problem could be handled without care, not knowing where to go for care, and not having the time to go for care.

Table 3. Key Barriers That May Hinder Veterans from Accessing Mental Health Care from VA

Key barrier	Description
Stigma and beliefs about mental health care	Veterans may have: • Perceptions that as a result of accessing mental health care they will be viewed negatively by others, such as peers or employers. For example, veterans may feel that by accessing mental health care they will be perceived as weak or having lost control. • Confidentiality and privacy concerns. For example, veterans may fear that accessing mental health care would harm their current or future careers. • Values and priorities—such as family, work, or school commitments—that conflict with accessing treatment. • Perceptions that treatment may bring up painful or trauma-related feelings and memories they wish to avoid. • Perceptions that social networks—such as families or military communities— have values and priorities that conflict with accessing treatment.
Lack of understanding or awareness of mental health care	Veterans may have: • Lack of knowledge about VA's mental health services. • Lack of awareness or understanding of their mental health conditions. For example, veterans may have difficulty distinguishing their mental health symptoms from the symptoms they are experiencing as a result of physical injuries. • Perception that mental health treatment is only for people with extreme mental health conditions. Veterans may feel that their mental health conditions are not severe enough to warrant treatment or that resources should go to those most in need. • Perception that mental health treatment is unnecessary or unhelpful.
Logistical challenges to accessing mental health care	Veterans may have: • Difficulty scheduling appointments. For example, veterans may have challenges coordinating multiple appointments or perceptions that there is limited availability of appointments. • Distance and transportation challenges. For example, veterans who live in rural areas may have to travel long distances to obtain treatment. • Family challenges, such as arranging child care or spousal support. • Other logistical challenges, such as time constraints or physical or mental impairments that may limit the opportunity to obtain treatment.
Concerns about VA's health care	Veterans may have: • Perceptions that VA's programs and service options are not adequate to meet their needs, such as not having enough providers or not having enough time during appointments to discuss both health and mental health care needs. • Perceptions that VA's services are not uniform across all provider locations (e.g., certain programs are not available at all VA medical centers). • Perceptions that VA's services are primarily or only for someone else, such as older veterans, war veterans, male veterans, or veterans with severe disabilities. • Perceptions that VA does not provide quality care to veterans, does not treat ve-terans well, or is not welcoming to particular groups of veterans (e.g., women). • Reluctance to talk with a VA mental health provider. For example, veterans may distrust mental health providers or fear that providers will not understand or believe them. • Negative perceptions about the government or VA.

Source: GAO's review of relevant literature published on or between January 1, 2006, and March 3, 2011, and corroborated by interviews with VA and VSO officials.

Additionally, according to the literature we reviewed and VA and VSO officials we interviewed, some of these key barriers may affect veterans from different demographic groups differently. For example, veterans may be affected by barriers differently based on age, gender, Reservist or National Guard status, or rural location.

- **Age**: OEF/OIF veterans, who are generally younger than other veterans, may have concerns about VA's health care system because they perceive that primarily older veterans, such as those who served in Vietnam, go to VA for care.[16] Additionally, some younger veterans may have multiple personal priorities—such as family, school, or work commitments—that make accessing care a lower priority. Older veterans may have different reasons for not accessing mental health care. For example, stigma and beliefs about mental health care may hinder veterans who served in World War II and Korea from accessing care because they grew up during a time when mental health conditions generally were not recognized and accepted. According to a national survey of veterans, as of March 2010, more than 60 percent of all veterans were 55 years of age or older.[17]

- **Gender**: Female veterans may perceive some barriers to accessing mental health care differently than male veterans.[18] For example, some female veterans may not identify themselves as veterans if they did not serve in combat and, as a result, may not access care from VA. In addition, female veterans may have concerns about VA's health care system because they perceive that the care is male oriented, and therefore, VA is not a place where they feel comfortable receiving mental health care. Female veterans are a growing demographic in the veteran population—from fiscal year 2010 to fiscal year 2020, the percentage of female veterans in the total veteran population is projected to increase from approximately 8 percent to approximately 10 percent, according to VA's National Center for Veterans Analysis and Statistics.[19] (See app. III for data on the gender of veterans receiving care from VA.)
- **Reservist or National Guard status**: Reservists and National Guard members may be particularly hindered by privacy and confidentiality concerns because they worry that accessing mental health care might have a negative impact on their military or civilian careers.[20] For example, Reservists and National Guard members may not access mental health care because of concerns about military leaders obtaining access to their VA health records and these leaders treating them differently or limiting their career development because they accessed mental health care. As of November 2010, Reservists and National Guard members made up nearly 50 percent of the OEF/OIF veteran population, according to VA data.
- **Rural location**: Veterans who live in rural locations may be particularly hindered by access challenges because of the distance they may have to travel to obtain mental health care.[21] According to the Office of Rural Health, veterans in rural areas are less likely to access mental health services than veterans in urban areas in part because they must travel greater distances to receive care and have more limited public transportation options. According to VA's Office of Rural Health, as of fiscal year 2010, veterans living in rural areas made up 41 percent of the veterans enrolled in VA's health care system.

VA Has Implemented Several Efforts to Increase Veterans' Access to Mental Health Care

VA has expanded options to increase veterans' access to mental health care and implemented education efforts to help connect veterans with care, according to VA officials.

VA Has Expanded Options to Increase Veterans' Access to Mental Health Care

VA has begun integrating mental health care into its primary care settings. Specifically, VA now requires its primary care clinics to conduct mental health screenings and has placed mental health care providers in primary care settings. For example, VA requires veterans treated in primary care settings to be screened for PTSD, depression, substance abuse disorders, and history of military sexual trauma.[22] Further, in 2008, VA began requiring primary care clinics that serve more than 1,500 veterans annually to have mental health providers available on-site, able to serve veterans.[23] Historically, veterans were more limited in the ways they could access VA's mental health services. For example, some veterans could receive mental health care only if they went to specialty VA mental health facilities, such as mental health clinics. According to VA, from fiscal years 2008 through 2010, the number of unique patients receiving mental health care in a primary care setting doubled. Several VA officials who work in primary care clinics that have integrated primary and mental health care told us that this integration is critical for lowering the stigma of receiving mental health care and for creating an environment of collaboration among providers for discussing veterans' needs and treatment options.

VA also has continued to increase the number of its Vet Centers, which provide confidential and free counseling services to address mental health issues. From fiscal year 2008 to August 2011, VA increased the number of Vet Centers from 232 to 292 and, according to VA, plans to open another 8 before the end of 2011. VA also has expanded the availability of Vet Center services through the use of approximately 70 Mobile Vet Centers—specially equipped vehicles that help bring Vet Center counseling services to more veterans, particularly those in rural areas. Vet Centers are often the first point of contact within VA for veterans and, according to VA and VSO officials, can help veterans overcome barriers to accessing mental health care. For example, many Vet Center counselors have firsthand combat experience, which, according to VA, helps them relate to veterans and reduce the stigma of mental health care that veterans may experience.

Additionally, VA has expanded its use of call centers to help connect veterans with counseling services. VA call centers are telephone-based systems through which veterans can access free, confidential counseling services. VA officials said that the call centers are an effective way to reach veterans because discussions with call center staff, many of whom are also veterans, may help callers assess whether they could benefit from mental health care. One call center VA operates, the Veterans Crisis Line, allows veterans and their families to call to receive multiple services, including suicide prevention services, 24 hours a day, 7 days a week.[24] According to VA officials, since the Veterans Crisis Line became operational in 2007, it has received more than 400,000 calls and referred approximately 55,000 veterans to local VA suicide prevention coordinators for same-day or next-day services. In addition to the Veterans Crisis Line, VA officials told us that VA has call centers focused on specific populations, such as combat veterans, homeless veterans, and family members of veterans.

Moreover, VA has increased its mental health staff from about 14,000 in fiscal year 2006 to more than 21,000 in fiscal year 2011, according to VA.[25] VA also has expanded the availability of telemental health services, which allow veterans to access mental health care providers remotely through VA medical centers, community-based outpatient clinics, and Mobile Vet Centers. Without telemental health, according to VA, some veterans in rural areas would have to drive as much as 5 hours to the nearest mental health provider, potentially decreasing their access to mental health care. To increase the availability of mental health appointments, as of 2007, VA required its mental health clinics to begin providing "after hours" treatment times, such as early morning, evening, or Saturday morning treatment times, to better accommodate veterans' schedules, including weekday school or work schedules. Additionally, as of 2007, VA has required that all veterans with mental health referrals be contacted within 24 hours to assess their needs; for nonemergency situations, VA requires that veterans receive follow-up care within 14 days of their referral.[26]

VA Has Implemented Education Efforts to Help Connect Veterans with Mental Health Care

To help connect veterans with mental health care, VA has implemented various efforts to educate veterans, veterans' families, health care providers, and other community stakeholders about mental health conditions and care. VA's efforts to help connect veterans with mental health care include collaborations with the Department of Defense, redesigned websites, and other technology-based education tools. VA has collaborated with the Department of Defense to educate veterans and active duty servicemembers returning home from deployments about VA benefits, including mental health care, through activities such as Yellow Ribbon Program events and postdeployment health reassessments.[27]

According to VA officials, VA has redesigned some of its key mental health websites—including its websites for the Office of Mental Health Services and the National Center for PTSD—to raise awareness of and provide convenient access to some of VA's mental health services, such as its call centers and resources for locating mental health providers. VA also has developed interactive technology-based tools to help educate veterans about how to recognize the symptoms of mental health conditions and connect with VA mental health care, including web-based self-help applications, mobile phone applications, and social media sites, such as Twitter and Facebook. In addition, VA has developed tailored efforts to educate specific groups of veterans, such as Native American veterans and veterans with serious mental illness. (See table 4 for examples of VA efforts to educate specific groups of veterans.)

VA also has efforts to educate veterans' families about what veterans may be experiencing and how to recognize the possible need for mental health care, according to VA officials. For example, VA has a guide for family members posted on its websites that describes common reactions to being in war, warning signs that a veteran or servicemember might need outside help, and where to go for help. According to VA and VSO officials, veterans' families are often the first to notice that the veteran is having mental health problems and may be more successful in encouraging the veteran to seek care.

Additionally, VA has trainings to teach its primary care physicians how to screen veterans for mental health conditions and have discussions with veterans about what to expect during mental health care. VA also has trainings for its providers covering topics such as the assessment and treatment of PTSD or military sexual trauma. According to VA, these types of trainings are important because primary care physicians are often a first point of contact for veterans who might benefit from VA mental health care. Additionally, the trainings help educate mental health care providers about evidence-based mental health practices, including issues regarding gender differences and cultural competencies. For example, according to VA, its National Center for PTSD offers web-based training intended to enhance VA staff sensitivity to, and knowledge of, specific health care needs affecting women veterans.[28]

VA also has developed efforts to educate other community stakeholders, including law enforcement personnel, chaplains, and employers, about veterans' mental health conditions and VA mental health care. For example, VA has a program that helps law enforcement personnel identify veterans with mental health conditions and connect these veterans to appropriate mental health treatment options. The literature shows that some veterans' mental health conditions have been found to increase their likelihood of entering or reentering the criminal justice system.[29] VA also has developed a series of training conferences for chaplains and clergy to educate them to recognize the symptoms of PTSD and other service-related mental health conditions and to refer veterans to VA for care. According to VA, training chaplains and clergy to recognize the symptoms of mental health conditions is important because they are often a first point of contact for veterans in need of assistance.

To support employers who may interact with veterans who have mental health conditions, VA has developed a set of online resources, including information on postdeployment mental health issues and information on mental health care available through VA.

Table 4. Examples of VA Efforts to Educate Specific Groups of Veterans about VA Mental Health Care

Specific group of veterans	Description of VA efforts
Native American veterans	Face-to-face outreach activities, including visits with tribal councils. Trainings for VA staff about how to conduct outreach that is culturally sensitive and focused specifically on the needs of Native American veterans.
Veterans with serious mental illness	Program to identify and reengage veterans with serious mental illness, such as schizophrenia, who have discontinued VA treatment.
Homeless veterans	Educational outreach and interventions in community locations, such as shelters and bus stations, to help eligible homeless veterans access VA benefits and care. Regional Stand Down events that provide information and services to homeless veterans, including health screenings that help identify potential mental health conditions and referrals to VA mental health care.
Reservists and National Guard members	VA staff presentations about eligibility for VA benefits, including mental health care, to Reservists and National Guard members at military bases.
Women veterans	Outreach to women using websites and brochures describing VA's specialized mental health care for women, such as women-only support groups to help women veterans who have experienced military sexual trauma. [a]
Student veterans	Outreach about VA's mental health services on college and university campuses to veterans enrolled as students.

Source: GAO analysis of VA data.

[a] Military sexual trauma includes both sexual harassment and sexual assault occurring during a servicemember's military career.

AGENCY COMMENTS

We provided a draft of this report to VA for comment. In its response, VA provided technical comments, which we have incorporated as appropriate.

Sincerely yours,

Debra A. Draper
Director, Health Care

APPENDIX I. SCOPE AND METHODOLOGY

To determine how many veterans received mental health care from the Department of Veterans Affairs (VA) from fiscal years 2006 through 2010, we obtained data from VA's Northeast Program Evaluation Center (NEPEC).[30] NEPEC used VA's administrative data files, which include inpatient and outpatient files, to generate counts of the number of veterans who received mental health care. For the purposes of this report, we defined mental health care as the care provided to veterans with mental health conditions. A veteran was counted as having a mental health condition if, at any point in the fiscal year, his or her medical record indicated at least two outpatient encounters with any mental health diagnosis (with at least one encounter having a primary mental health diagnosis) or an inpatient stay in which the veteran had any mental health diagnosis.[31] Additionally, the number of veterans represents a unique count of veterans; veterans were counted only once, even if they received care multiple times during a fiscal year or across the 5-year period. NEPEC also used VA administrative data files to provide us with data on the total number of veterans receiving any health care at VA—not just veterans receiving mental health care. The number of veterans includes former active duty servicemembers, including Reservists and National Guard members.[32]

NEPEC's data on the number of veterans receiving mental health care included breakouts by specific demographic groups, such as era of service; by the type of setting where care was provided; and by the mental health diagnostic category. For the era of service data, NEPEC identified two groups of veterans: (1) veterans serving in the Operations Enduring Freedom (OEF) and Iraqi Freedom (OIF) era and (2) veterans from all other eras—including peacetime. Because OEF/OIF veterans are not tracked separately from Persian Gulf War veterans in VA's administrative data files, NEPEC used Department of Defense data to identify OEF/OIF veterans from the total population of veterans in the VA data. The non-OEF/OIF veterans in the VA data comprised the veterans from all other eras. Veterans who served in more than one era of service were assigned based on their most recent era of service. NEPEC also provided data on the settings where care was provided—that is, specialty mental health care settings that primarily provided mental health services or other settings that may have provided some mental health services but focus primarily on other types of care, such as primary care. Furthermore, NEPEC provided data on the top five mental health diagnostic categories.[33] The most common diagnostic categories were determined based on the number of veterans with diagnoses included in the diagnostic category, not the number of visits associated with the diagnoses. To assess the reliability of the data NEPEC provided us, we discussed with NEPEC officials their methodology and data collection techniques used for obtaining and using the data, the data checks that NEPEC performed, as well as any limitations officials identified in the data. In addition, we did our own review of NEPEC's programming and methodological approaches using data file documentation, code book and file dictionaries, and programming logs NEPEC officials provided. We determined that the data were sufficiently reliable for our purposes. The data on veterans receiving care from VA are not necessarily representative of the entire veteran population because some veterans receive care outside of VA.

To identify the key barriers that may hinder veterans from accessing mental health care from VA, we searched research databases, such as MEDLINE and PsycINFO, that included peer-reviewed journals to capture relevant literature published on or between January 1, 2006, and March 3, 2011. We searched these databases for articles with key words in their titles or subject terms related to veterans, mental health, and barriers. In addition, we also reviewed relevant literature that was cited in articles from our original search or recommended to us during the course of our research. To corroborate the barriers identified in the literature, we interviewed officials from (1) several VA offices—the Office of Mental Health Services, the Office of Mental Health Operations, the Office of Rural Health, the Office of Research and Development, and Readjustment Counseling Services; (2) several mental health–focused VA research centers—the Mental Illness Research, Education and Clinical Center, the Serious Mental Illness Treatment Resource and Evaluation Center, the Center for Chronic Disease Outcomes Research, and the National Center for PTSD; (3) several VA mental health and primary care providers;[34] and (4) a judgmental sample of veterans service organizations (VSO).[35] We defined "key barriers" as those that the majority of VA and VSO officials we interviewed said could have the greatest impact on veterans. As a result, we do not report an exhaustive list of all possible barriers that veterans may face.

To identify the efforts VA has implemented to increase veterans' access to VA mental health care, we interviewed officials from the same VA offices and mental health–focused VA research centers that we interviewed to corroborate the barriers for veterans. We also reviewed supporting VA documentation, such as program descriptions, policy directives, and congressional budget justifications. We compiled a list of efforts by focusing on the efforts that had been implemented and were national in scope. As a result, the list of efforts we report is not an exhaustive list of all VA efforts. In addition, we did not assess the extent to which VA has fully implemented these efforts or their effectiveness, including the extent to which the efforts eliminate or diminish barriers that may hinder veterans from accessing mental health care.

We conducted our work from November 2010 to October 2011 in accordance with all sections of GAO's Quality Assurance Framework that are relevant to our objectives. The framework requires that we plan and perform the engagement to obtain sufficient and appropriate evidence to meet our stated objectives and to discuss any limitations in our work. We believe that the information and data obtained, and the analysis conducted, provide a reasonable basis for any findings and conclusions.

Appendix II. Number of Veterans Receiving Mental Health Care from VA by Setting and Era, Fiscal Years 2006 through 2010

Era of military service	2006		2007		2008		2009		2010	
	Specialty mental health care setting	Other settings	Specialty mental health care setting	Other settings	Specialty mental health care setting	Other settings	Specialty mental health care setting	Other settings	Specialty mental health care setting	Other settings
OEF/OIF	32,235	33,123	52,037	53,164	78,693	81,339	105,628	109,865	129,399	134,970
All other eras of service	701,988	845,067	733,129	881,287	777,718	928,956	829,792	991,306	885,230	1,049,819
Total	**734,223**	**878,190**	**785,166**	**934,451**	**856,411**	**1,010,295**	**935,420**	**1,101,171**	**1,014,629**	**1,184,789**

Source: NEPEC.

Notes: Specialty mental health settings, including mental health clinics, primarily provide mental health services. Other settings may provide some mental health services but focus primarily on other types of care, such as primary care. The numbers do not add to the total number of veterans receiving mental health care because veterans may have received care in both types of settings. Additionally, the number of veterans represents a unique count of veterans; veterans were counted only once, even if they received care multiple times during a fiscal year or multiple times in each type of setting.

Appendix III. Number of Veterans Receiving Care from VA by Gender and Era, Fiscal Years 2006 through 2010

Era of military service	2006		2007		2008		2009		2010	
	Male	**Female**	**Male**	**Female**	**Male**	**Female**	**Male**	**Female**	**Male**	**Female**
Veterans receiving mental health care from VA										
OEF/ OIF	29,842	4,717	48,379	6,964	73,776	10,171	99,904	13,373	122,428	16,739
All other eras of service	800,334	62,236	830,415	66,904	871,230	72,815	924,566	80,803	975,983	88,380
Total	**830,176**	**66,953**	**878,794**	**73,868**	**945,006**	**82,986**	**1,024,470**	**94,176**	**1,098,411**	**105,119**
All veterans receiving any health care from VA										
OEF/OIF	127,821	19,239	174,644	25,313	223,975	32,266	280,643	39,190	338,737	47,789
All other eras of service	4,424,742	217,539	4,406,149	224,458	4,395,448	232,561	4,465,169	245,299	4,589,963	260,006
Total	**4,552,563**	**236,778**	**4,580,793**	**249,771**	**4,619,423**	**264,827**	**4,745,812**	**284,489**	**4,928,700**	**307,795**

Source: NEPEC.

Note: The number of veterans represents a unique count of veterans; veterans were counted only once, even if they received care multiple times during a fiscal year.

End Notes

[1] Veterans who served in active military and who were discharged or released under conditions other than dishonorable are generally eligible for VA health care. Reservists and National Guard members may also be eligible for VA health care if they were called to active duty by a federal order and completed the full period for which they were called. Veterans can also receive health care funded by sources other than VA, including private insurance, Medicare, and Medicaid. In general, veterans must enroll in VA health care to receive VA's medical benefits package—a set of services that includes a full range of hospital and outpatient services, prescription drugs, and noninstitutional long-term care services.

[2] Military operations in Afghanistan occurring after September 2010 are referred to as Operation New Dawn. For the purposes of this report, we refer to all veterans participating in military operations in Afghanistan as OEF veterans.

[3] See 38 U.S.C. § 1710(a), 38 C.F.R. §§ 17.36, 17.38 (2009). Any veteran who has served in a combat theater after November 11, 1998, including OEF/OIF veterans, and who was discharged or released from active service on or after January 28, 2003, has up to 5 years from the date of the veteran's most recent discharge or release from active duty service to enroll in VA's health care system and receive VA health care services. See 38 U.S.C. § 1710(e)(1)(D), (e)(3).

[4] See GAO, *VA Health Care: Reporting of Spending and Workload for Mental Health Services Could Be Improved*, GAO-10-570 (Washington, D.C.: May 28, 2010).

[5] NEPEC is one of VA's national evaluation centers, and it evaluates and monitors the mental health care delivered by VA nationally.

[6] Because providers may document a mental health diagnosis while providing care for a non–mental health condition, a portion of this care may be unrelated to a mental health condition.

[7] The mental health and primary care providers we spoke with were identified by VA officials as having specific knowledge of either barriers to veterans accessing mental health care or efforts VA has implemented to increase veterans' access to VA mental health care.

[8] We spoke with officials from eight VSOs: American Legion, American Veterans, Disabled American Veterans, Paralyzed Veterans of America, Veterans of Modern Warfare, Vietnam Veterans of America, Women Veterans of America, and Wounded Warrior Project.

[9] The Veterans' Health Care Eligibility Reform Act of 1996, Pub. L. No. 104-262, 110 Stat. 3177, 3182, § 104 (Oct. 9, 1996), codified at 38 U.S.C. § 1705, directed VA to establish a patient enrollment system to manage the provision of care and services by establishing priority groups and directing VA to enroll veterans in accordance with the priorities.

[10] For example, in fiscal year 2010 approximately 790,000 veterans were identified as having service-connected mental health disorder disabilities.

[11] See 38 U.S.C. § 101.

[12] The number of veterans receiving care from VA includes eligible former active duty servicemembers, including Reservists and National Guard members. In some cases, VA also provides care to nonveterans, such as active duty servicemembers or veterans' dependents; however, nonveterans were not included in our analysis. Veterans who received care were counted only once, even if they received care multiple times during a fiscal year or across the 5-year period.

[13] In fiscal year 2010, about 1 million veterans received mental health care in specialty mental health care settings and about 1.2 million veterans received mental health care in other settings. These numbers do not add to the total number of veterans receiving mental health care in fiscal year 2010 because veterans may have received care in both types of settings.

[14] Among the general U.S. population, an estimated 26 percent of adults experience a mental health condition in a given year. See R.C. Kessler, W.T. Chiu, O. Demler, K.R. Merikangas, and E.E. Walters, "Prevalence, Severity, and Comorbidity of 12-Month DSMIV Disorders in the National Comorbidity Survey Replication," *Archives of General Psychiatry*, vol. 62, no. 6 (2005).

[15] Substance Abuse and Mental Health Services Administration, Office of Applied Studies, *Results from the 2008 National Survey on Drug Use and Health*, NSDUH Series H-36, HHS Publication No. SMA 09-4434 (Rockville, Md.: September 2009).

[16] See for example, M. A. Burnam et al., "Mental Health Care for Iraq and Afghanistan War Veterans," *Health Affairs*, vol. 28, no. 3 (2009).

[17] Westat, *The National Survey of Veterans, Active Duty Service Members, Demobilized National Guard and Reserve Members, Family Members and Surviving Spouses*, prepared for the Department of Veterans Affairs (Rockville, Md.: Oct. 18, 2010).

[18] See for example, A. E. Street, D. Vogt, and L. Dutra, "A New Generation of Women Veterans: Stressors Faced by Women Deployed to Iraq and Afghanistan," *Clinical Psychology Review*, vol. 29, no. 8 (2009).

[19] Department of Veterans Affairs, National Center for Veterans Analysis and Statistics, *Veteran Population Projections: FY2000 to FY2036* (December 2010).

[20] See, for example, C.S. Milliken, J.L. Auchterlonie, and C.W. Hoge, "Longitudinal Assessment of Mental Health Problems Among Active and Reserve Component Soldiers Returning From the Iraq War," *JAMA*, vol. 298, no. 18 (2007).

[21] See, for example, A. West and W.B. Weeks, "Physical and Mental Health and Access to Care Among Nonmetropolitan Veterans Health Administration Patients Younger than 65 Years," *Journal of Rural Health*, vol. 22, no. 1 (2006).

[22] Military sexual trauma includes both sexual harassment and sexual assault occurring during a servicemember's military career. VA is required to operate a program to provide counseling and treatment for veterans suffering from sexual trauma under 38 U.S.C. § 1720D.

[23] Primary care clinics in facilities that serve fewer than 1,500 veterans can provide access to mental health professionals who may not be on-site, through options such as telemental health services.

[24] The Veterans Crisis Line (1-800-273-TALK) was established as a partnership between VA, the Substance Abuse and Mental Health Services Administration, and the National Suicide Prevention Lifeline. Callers to this call center talk to trained counselors about their concerns and can be referred to VA mental health service providers in their area, or receive emergency interventions if necessary. This service is also available to veterans who visit the program's website (http://www.veteranscrisisline.net/) through online chat services. The Veterans Crisis Line is part of VA's Suicide Prevention Program. In addition to the Veterans Crisis Line, VA's Suicide Prevention Program also includes national outreach campaigns to educate the public about suicide prevention and local suicide prevention coordinators who provide information to veterans in their communities.

[25] According to VA officials, these mental health staff include mental health providers, such as psychiatrists, psychologists, and social workers, as well as additional staff, such as occupational therapists and pharmacists.

[26] Also in 2007, VA required its emergency rooms to have mental health staff available for consultation 24 hours a day, 7 days a week, and for its urgent care centers to have mental health providers available during their hours of operation.

[27] The Yellow Ribbon Program is a Department of Defense effort to help Reservists and National Guard members and their families connect with local resources, including information on VA mental health care, especially during the reintegration phase that occurs months after servicemembers return home. Postdeployment health reassessments are a Department of Defense program for assessing the physical and mental health condition of servicemembers from 90 to 180 days after deployment. During these events, VA officials are present to help with enrollment in VA health care and to provide referrals, as necessary, for mental health care.

[28] The National Center for PTSD is one of VA's Centers of Excellence, or communities of researchers and educational professionals focused on certain mental health issues. According to VA officials, this center identifies best practices through research, participates in the development of clinical practice guidelines describing best practices, and works to disseminate them through educational programs for VA mental health providers to use, among other activities.

[29] For example, see H. Balshem, V. Christensen, A. Tuepker, and D. Kansagara, *A Critical Review of the Literature Regarding Homelessness among Veterans*, VA-ESP Project #05- 225 (2011).

[30] NEPEC is one of VA's national evaluation centers, and it evaluates and monitors the mental health care delivered by VA nationally.

[31] Because providers may document a mental health diagnosis while providing care for a non-mental health condition, a portion of this care may be unrelated to a mental health condition.

[32] The number of veterans does not include veterans who only received medications, or contract, or fee-based care. Contract and fee-based care represent inpatient and outpatient care, respectively, that VA may authorize veterans to receive at non-VA health care facilities. VA also provides care to nonveterans such as active duty servicemembers and veterans' dependents; however, nonveterans were not included in our analysis.

[33] NEPEC uses standardized diagnostic categories that include specific International Classification of Diseases, Ninth Revision, codes for mental health diagnoses.

[34] The mental health and primary care providers we spoke with were identified by VA officials as having specific knowledge of either barriers to veterans accessing mental health care or efforts VA has implemented to increase veterans' access to VA mental health care.

[35] We spoke with officials from eight VSOs: American Legion, American Veterans, Disabled American Veterans, Paralyzed Veterans of America, Veterans of Modern Warfare, Vietnam Veterans of America, Women Veterans of America, and Wounded Warrior Project.

In: Veteran Injuries, Disorders and Medical Care Service ISBN: 978-1-62081-302-7
Editors: Jessica Michaels and Jesse E. Levine

Chapter 7

VA Community Living Centers: Actions Needed to Better Manage Risks to Veterans' Quality of Life and Care*

United States Government Accountability Office

Why GAO Did This Study

The Department of Veterans Affairs (VA) annually provides care to more than 46,000 elderly and disabled veterans in 132 VA-operated nursing homes, called community living centers (CLC). After media reports of problems with the care delivered to veterans in CLCs, VA contracted with the Long Term Care Institute, Inc. (LTCI), a nonprofit organization that surveys nursing homes, to conduct in-depth reviews of CLCs in 2007-2008 and again in 2010-2011. GAO was asked to evaluate VA's approach to managing veterans' quality of care and quality of life in CLCs. This report examines (1) VA's response to and resolution of LTCI-identified deficiencies and (2) information VA collects about the quality of care and quality of life in CLCs and how VA uses it to identify and manage risks. To do this work, GAO interviewed officials from VA headquarters, examined all 116 2007-2008 and 67 2010-2011 LTCI reviews, and analyzed 50 CLCs' corrective action plans for 2007-2008 and 23 such plans for 2010-2011.

What GAO Recommends

GAO recommends that VA document feedback to CLCs and require periodic status reports about corrective action plan implementation, and implement a process to comprehensively identify and manage risks to residents in CLCs by analyzing and comparing information about residents' quality of care and quality of life. In its comments on a draft of this report, VA concurred with these recommendations.

* This is an edited, reformatted and augmented version of the Highlights of GAO-12-11, a report to the Ranking Member, Committee on Veterans' Affairs, U.S. Senate, dated October 2011.

WHAT GAO FOUND

VA headquarters established a process for responding to deficiencies identified at CLCs during the 2007 and 2008 LTCI reviews. VA is using the process, which requires CLCs to submit corrective action plans addressing LTCI-identified deficiencies—such as how CLCs will address a lack of competent nursing staff and a failure to provide a sanitary and safe living environment—during the 2010 and 2011 LTCI reviews. On the basis of its analysis of the deficiencies identified in 2007 and 2008, VA headquarters also developed a national training and education initiative. VA headquarters officials told GAO that they plan to analyze the deficiencies identified during the 2010 and 2011 reviews and identify national areas for improvement. However, GAO found weaknesses in VA's process for responding to and resolving LTCI-identified deficiencies. First, VA headquarters does not maintain clear and complete documentation of the feedback it provides to CLCs regarding their corrective action plans. Second, VA headquarters does not require VA's networks, which oversee the operations of VA medical facilities, including CLCs, to report on the status of CLCs' implementation of corrective action plans or to verify CLCs' self-reported compliance with the requirements of the national training and education initiative. Because of these weaknesses, VA headquarters cannot provide reasonable assurance that LTCI-identified deficiencies are resolved. For example, without requiring networks to report on the status of CLCs' implementation of their corrective action plans, VA headquarters cannot determine whether CLCs' corrective action plans are fully implemented. Unaddressed, weaknesses in VA headquarters' process for responding to LTCI-identified deficiencies may compromise the quality of care and quality of life of veterans in CLCs.

VA headquarters' current approach to identifying risks associated with the quality of care and quality of life of CLC residents does not comprehensively analyze information from all available sources, and for the sources VA does analyze, it does not compare findings across sources. VA's approach relies significantly on the analysis of findings from LTCI reviews of CLCs. However, in addition to LTCI reviews, VA headquarters obtains information about CLCs from a variety of other sources, such as VA's Office of Inspector General (OIG), but does not analyze the information from all these other sources. Further, for the sources it does analyze, VA headquarters evaluates each source in isolation and does not compare the findings from one source with findings from the other sources. Therefore, VA headquarters' current approach to identifying risks in CLCs may result in missed opportunities to detect patterns and trends in information about the quality of care and quality of life within a CLC or across many CLCs. For example, in comparing findings from VA's Office of the Medical Inspector, OIG, LTCI, and VA's quality indicator and quality measure data for one CLC, GAO found a pattern of deficiencies related to pain management. Without considering information from all available sources and comparing it across sources, VA headquarters cannot fully identify risks in CLCs, estimate the significance of the risks, or take actions to mitigate them.

ABBREVIATIONS

CLC	community living center
LTCI	Long Term Care Institute, Inc.
OIG	Office of Inspector General
OMI	Office of the Medical Inspector
PICC	peripherally inserted central catheter
SOARS	System-wide Ongoing Assessment and Review Strategy
VA	Department of Veterans Affairs
VAMC	VA medical center

October 19, 2011

The Honorable Richard Burr
Ranking Member
Committee on Veterans' Affairs
United States Senate
Dear Senator Burr:

The Department of Veterans Affairs (VA) spent more than $4.5 billion on nursing home care in fiscal year 2010, over $3.3 billion of which was for care in 132 VA-operated nursing homes, called community living centers (CLC).[1] CLCs offer a range of services that include short-term postacute rehabilitation for conditions such as a stroke; long-term care for veterans who cannot be cared for at home because of severe and chronic physical or mental limitations; and end-of-life care for terminal illnesses. More than 46,000 elderly and disabled veterans annually receive care in CLCs. This vulnerable population relies on VA to ensure they receive quality care and maintain their quality of life while residing in a CLC.[2]

In 2004, problems related to the care and conditions in one CLC surfaced in the media, raising concerns about the effectiveness of VA's efforts to manage the quality of care and quality of life in its CLCs. In response, VA headquarters had in-depth unannounced reviews conducted at selected CLCs between August 2004 and November 2006, and contracted with the Long Term Care Institute, Inc. (LTCI), in March 2007 to conduct in-depth reviews of 116 CLCs.[3] LTCI conducted its reviews between June 2007 and September 2008.[4] In late 2009, a series of newspaper articles reported the details of deficiencies that LTCI had identified at another CLC in September 2008. Specifically, the articles reported a lack of competent skilled nursing in the CLC as well as failure to provide a sanitary and safe living environment, promote and protect veterans' rights to autonomy, and treat veterans with respect and dignity.

Recognizing the value of the information obtained from the in-depth reviews of CLCs, VA headquarters awarded a second contract in July 2010 to LTCI to begin reviewing all 132 CLCs in September 2010. In light of this contract and the 2009 newspaper articles, you raised questions about VA's process for responding to the deficiencies identified during the LTCI reviews, as well as the agency's overall approach to managing the quality of care and quality of life in its CLCs. These questions included how VA headquarters uses available information regarding the quality of care and quality of life in its CLCs, such as the deficiencies cited by LTCI, to identify patterns and associated risks and take appropriate actions to address those risks. This report examines (1) actions VA headquarters has taken to respond to and resolve LTCI-identified deficiencies and (2) what information VA headquarters collects regarding the quality of care and quality of life in CLCs and the extent to which VA headquarters uses the information to identify and manage risks.

To examine actions VA headquarters has taken to respond to and resolve deficiencies LTCI identified during its 2007 and 2008, and 2010 and 2011, reviews of CLCs, we obtained and analyzed copies of the 116 LTCI reviews performed during 2007 and 2008; VA headquarters' subsequent analyses of those reviews; copies of 50 CLCs' corrective action plans and related documentation from the 2007 and 2008 reviews;[5] copies of the 67 LTCI reviews performed between September 1, 2010, and March 31, 2011; and copies of 23 CLCs' corrective action plans from the 2010 and 2011 reviews.[6] We also reviewed relevant VA policy documents, including Veterans Health Administration Directive 2009-43, Quality Management System. We interviewed officials from VA headquarters offices involved in responding to LTCI-identified deficiencies, including the Office of Geriatrics and Extended Care and the Office of the Deputy Under Secretary for Health for Operations and Management.[7] In addition, we reviewed Executive Career Field Plans of VA network directors and interviewed officials from 2 of VA's 21 networks, which oversee the operations of the various medical facilities within their assigned geographic area. These two networks were the VA Mid-Atlantic Health Care Network (Durham, North Carolina) and the VA Northwest Health Network (Vancouver, Washington). To select the networks, we considered the average number of deficiencies per CLC reviewed by LTCI in 2007 and 2008.[8] We assessed VA headquarters' response to identified deficiencies in the context of federal standards for internal control for monitoring, control activities, and information and communications.[9] The internal control for monitoring refers to an agency's ability to provide reasonable assurance that actions are taken in response to the findings from reviews and the deficiencies identified are promptly resolved, while the internal control for control activities refers to an agency's ability to provide reasonable assurance that management's directives are carried out, which includes appropriately documenting transactions and internal controls. The internal control for information and communications refers to an agency's ability to provide reasonable assurance of the relevance and reliability of information necessary to achieve an agency's objectives, including verifying the accuracy of its data.

To determine what information VA headquarters collects regarding the quality of care and quality of life in CLCs and the extent to which VA headquarters uses the information to identify and manage risks, we reviewed reports from reviews and investigations performed at CLCs between June 2007 and June 2011. We also reviewed VA analyses of information contained in these reports and VA policy documents. We interviewed officials from Geriatrics and Extended Care; the Office of the Deputy Under Secretary for Health for Operations and Management; the Office of the Assistant Deputy Under Secretary for Health for Informatics and Analytics; the Office of the Assistant Deputy Under Secretary for Health for Quality, Safety, and Value; and the Office of Inspector General (OIG). We assessed VA headquarters' use of information regarding the quality of care and quality of life in CLCs in the context of federal standards for internal control for risk assessment. The internal control for risk assessment refers to an agency's ability to identify and analyze relevant risks associated with achieving its objectives.

We conducted this performance audit from August 2010 through September 2011 in accordance with generally accepted government auditing standards. Those standards require that we plan and perform the audit to obtain sufficient, appropriate evidence to provide a reasonable basis for our findings and conclusions based on our audit objectives. We believe that the evidence obtained provides a reasonable basis for our findings and conclusions based on our audit objectives.

BACKGROUND

VA provides nursing home care for some veterans, as required, and makes these services available to other veterans on a discretionary basis, as resources permit.[10] Specifically, VA is required by law to provide nursing home care to any veteran who needs it for a service-connected disability and to any veteran who needs it and has a service-connected disability rated at 70 percent or greater.[11] However, VA provides most of its nursing home care to veterans on a discretionary basis, as resources permit.[12] VA's policy on nursing home eligibility requires that VA networks provide nursing home care to veterans with 60 percent service-connected disability ratings who are either unemployable or who have been determined by VA to be permanently and totally disabled. For all other veterans, VA's policy is to provide nursing home care on a discretionary basis, with certain veterans having higher priority, including veterans who require care following a hospitalization.

CLCs provide both short-stay (90 days or less) and long-stay (more than 90 days) services. According to VA data, almost 94 percent of th residents admitted to CLCs in fiscal year 2010 were short-stay. Short-stay care in CLCs includes skilled nursing care, rehabilitation, restorative care maintenance care for those awaiting alternative placement, hospice, and respite care. The remaining admissions, about 6 percent, were long-stay. Long-stay care includes dementia care, maintenance care, and care for those with spinal cord injury and disorders.

Responsibility for VA's medical facilities, including CLCs, rests with both VA's networks and VA headquarters. Almost all of VA's 132 CLCs, located throughout VA's 21 networks, are colocated with or in close proximity to a VA medical center (VAMC). While networks are charged with the day-to-day management of the VAMCs within their network, VA headquarters maintains responsibility for establishing national policy and overseeing both networks and VAMC operations. Within VA headquarters, Geriatrics and Extended Care is responsible for developing VA's policies and other national actions related to the quality of care and quality of life in VA's CLCs. The Office of the Deputy Under Secretary for Health for Operations and Management, through each network, ensures that VAMCs, including CLCs, comply with VA's policies and implement other national actions.

The LTCI contract, which began in September 2010, is for 1 year, and provides for LTCI to conduct reviews between September 2010 and August 2011. VA may exercise an option to renew for each of 4 additional years through August 2015.[13] Officials from both Geriatrics and Extended Care and the Office of the Deputy Under Secretary for Health for Operations and Management share responsibility for administering VA's contract with LTCI.

LTCI uses the Centers for Medicare & Medicaid Services' scope and severity scale for classifying nursing home deficiencies. There are four severity classifications, with the least serious deficiencies rated as having the potential for minimal harm and the most serious deficiencies rated as immediate jeopardy situations—in which residents are potentially or actually at risk of dying or being seriously injured. The remaining two severity classifications are actual harm and potential for more than minimal harm. The scope of deficiencies—or the number of residents potentially or actually affected by the deficient care—may be rated as isolated, pattern, or widespread.

VA policy requires that all VAMCs be accredited by The Joint Commission.[14] As part of the accreditation process for a VAMC, which occurs on average every 3 years, The Joint Commission surveys and accredits any CLC associated with the VAMC.[15] VA requires CLCs to meet The Joint Commission long-term care standards.[16] CLCs are also subject to periodic reviews by VA's OIG.

VA Headquarters Established a Process for Responding to LTCI-Identified Deficiencies, but Cannot Provide Reasonable Assurance That Deficiencies Have been Resolved

VA headquarters established a process for responding to deficiencies identified at CLCs during the 2007 and 2008 reviews. This process, which requires CLCs to submit corrective action plans addressing LTCIidentified deficiencies—such as how CLCs will address a lack of competent nursing staff and a failure to provide a sanitary and safe living environment—is also being used during the 2010 and 2011 LTCI reviews. However, because of weaknesses in the process, VA headquarters cannot provide reasonable assurance that deficiencies that could potentially affect the quality of care and quality of life of residents are resolved.

VA Headquarters' Process Requires Corrective Action Plans and, for 2007 and 2008, National Training and Education

VA headquarters established a process for responding to LTCI-identified deficiencies that requires each CLC to develop a corrective action plan addressing all deficiencies identified and submit it to VA headquarters within 30 days of receiving an LTCI report. The plans may include actions such as training CLC staff on clinical policies and procedures or implementing nursing and interdisciplinary rounds to monitor the clinical issues related to the deficiencies. VA headquarters officials review each corrective action plan to determine whether the actions can be expected to correct all identified deficiencies and whether the time frames for completing the actions are reasonable. The officials then provide each CLC feedback by telephone, discussing any revisions to the corrective action plans that may be necessary. The officials document these discussions using hand-written notes on hard copies of CLCs' corrective action plans, which are not shared with VA networks and CLCs. VA headquarters officials told us they may schedule additional telephone calls with CLCs when significant revision of a corrective action plan is necessary or if the officials want an update on the implementation of the plan. For deficiencies identified in the 2007 and 2008 LTCI reviews, the documentation showed that officials had at least two telephone calls with 29 of the 116 CLCs reviewed.[17] Three of these 29 CLCs received more than two follow-up calls. When additional calls were made, VA headquarters required the CLCs to submit an updated corrective action plan.

Table 1. Clinical High-Risk Categories Defined by VA Headquarters' Analysis of Deficiencies Identified in 2007 and 2008 Long Term Care Institute, Inc., Reviews

Category	Percentage of 116 CLCs with related deficiencies[a]	Examples of deficiencies
Dignity	90	• Residents lacked privacy, including exposure during care; provision of care in public areas, such as applying ointment to a resident's upper body in the dining room in front of other residents; and uncovered catheter bags attached to residents' wheelchairs. • Residents had poor hygiene, including having dirty fingernails, not being shaven or bathed, and generally looking unkempt.
Medication management	78	• Residents were not assessed prior to administering medication (e.g., blood pressure not taken before administering hypertension medication or blood sugar testing not completed before administering insulin). • Medication was not administered according to policy and procedures. For example, staff did not document insulin injection sites or check documentation for prior insulin injection sites to ensure that insulin would not be injected routinely into the same site. Not rotating insulin injection sites can lead to hardening of the skin or weakening of fatty tissue under the skin. These can change the way insulin is absorbed, making it difficult to manage blood glucose levels.
Infection control	59	• Staff did not adhere to proper isolation procedures (e.g., entering and exiting rooms of residents with infectious diseases without wearing or removing protective gowns and gloves). • Staff did not follow handwashing policies and procedures.
Psychotropic medications[b]	47	• Staff administered psychotropic medications as a restraint and beyond the scope of the physician's original order (e.g., using psychotropic medications to calm residents before trying other nonpharmaco-logical interventions to manage behavior). • Staff did not track and review residents' behavior to help ensure that use of a psychotropic medication was appropriate.

Table 1. (Continued)

Category	Percentage of 116 CLCs with related deficiencies[a]	Examples of deficiencies
Percutaneous endoscopic gastrostomy tubes[c]	30	• Staff did not ensure full doses of medications were administered. • Residents experiencing significant weight loss were not assessed by a practitioner.
Restraints	28	• Staff were not trained to know which devices were classified as restraints and therefore used restraints without physician authorization (e.g., staff used bed rails, seat belts, and tables to restrict resident mobility, all of which are classified as restraints).
Pressure ulcers[d]	24	• Residents were not regularly assessed for having or being at risk for pressure ulcers. • Residents with pressure ulcers did not receive proper care, including wound care.
Peripherally inserted central catheter (PICC) lines[e]	21	• Staff did not properly prepare lines (e.g., did not flush lines) before and after administering medications, when required. • Staff did not follow procedures for dressing changes of PICC lines, which could increase the risk of local or systemic infection.

Source: Long Term Care Institute, Inc. (LTCI), and VA data.

Notes: GAO analyzed data contained in the 2007 and 2008 LTCI reviews and data provided by VA headquarters based on its analysis of the 2007 and 2008 LTCI reviews.

[a] Represents the percentage of 116 community living centers (CLC) where LTCI identified at least one deficiency related to that category in 2007 or 2008.

[b] A psychotropic medication is any medication whose intended purpose is to alter perception, mental status, or behavior. Examples of drug classes include antipsychotic, antidepressant, and antianxiety medications.

[c] A percutaneous endoscopic gastrostomy tube is a flexible feeding tube that is placed through the abdominal wall and into the stomach to allow nutrition, fluids, and medications to be put directly into the stomach.

[d] Pressure ulcers are areas of damaged skin caused by staying in one position for too long. They commonly form where bones are close to the skin, such as ankles, back, elbows, heels, and hips. Residents are at risk if they are bedridden, use a wheelchair, or are unable to change position. Pressure ulcers can lead to serious infections, some of which are life-threatening.

[e] A central line is a small tube that is placed in a large vein in the neck, chest, groin, or arm to give fluids, blood, or medications or to do medical tests quickly. A central line can remain for weeks or months, and some patients receive treatment through the line several times a day. A PICC line is a specific type of central line that is placed into a vein in the arm.

While VA's process requires that all deficiencies identified be addressed, it gives priority to deficiencies at the immediate jeopardy or actual harm levels. When LTCI review teams identify such deficiencies during a survey, they are required to notify VA headquarters and the relevant VAMC.[18] LTCI identified immediate jeopardy or actual harm deficiencies at 25 of the 116 CLCs (about 22 percent) reviewed in 2007 and 2008, and at 10 of the 67 CLCs (about 15 percent of the CLCs) reviewed in 2010 and 2011 as of March 31, 2011.[19]

After the 2007 and 2008 LTCI reviews, VA headquarters officials analyzed the deficiencies from the 116 reviews and from the analysis developed eight clinical high-risk categories. According to these officials, the eight categories, which included medication management, infection control, and peripherally inserted central catheter (PICC) lines, posed the greatest risk to residents' health and safety.[20] (See table 1.) The officials then implemented a national training and education initiative to address the eight categories.

VA headquarters convened a workgroup that developed national training guidelines and checklists for evaluating CLC staff competencies in each of the eight categories. The workgroup included representatives from Geriatrics and Extended Care, the Office of Nursing Services,[21] Nutrition and Food Services,[22] and the Infectious Diseases Program Office.[23] A VA headquarters official told us that the workgroup included the last three offices because the majority of LTCI-identified deficiencies were related to nursing, nutrition, and infection control issues. VA headquarters provided the VA networks and CLCs with the national guidelines and checklists and required CLCs to incorporate them into their training and education policies. VA headquarters required CLCs to report whether they had met the following four requirements for each of the eight clinical high-risk categories: (1) establish CLC policies, (2) adopt procedures for implementing the policies,[24] (3) design an assessment to observe staff proficiency in providing care matching the established procedure, and (4) establish a plan for ongoing training and assessment of staff, including new staff.[25] In addition, CLCs were required to directly observe staff providing care to CLC residents and report the percentage of staff that had been observed as being proficient in the procedures necessary to comply with CLCs' policies for each of the eight clinical high-risk categories.[26] If CLCs did not meet all four requirements for each category or had observed less than 90 percent of their staff as proficient in providing care in any one of the clinical high-risk categories, they were to develop and submit corrective action plans to VA headquarters. According to the documentation we reviewed, in most categories, the majority of CLCs indicated that they had met the requirements of the national training and education initiative. However, in every category there were CLCs that did not meet these requirements and had to submit a corrective action plan. For example, for the medication management clinical high-risk category, 14 of the 132 CLCs submitted a corrective action plan because they either were not in compliance with the four requirements or had not observed at least 90 percent of their staff as being proficient in providing care.[27]

After LTCI's 2010 and 2011 reviews of VA's CLCs are complete, VA headquarters plans to analyze the deficiencies identified by LTCI. To facilitate the analysis, VA headquarters is working with LTCI to track and note trends with regard to deficiencies on a quarterly basis. LTCI provides quarterly reports to VA headquarters, which include data on which deficiencies are the most frequently identified nationally. For each CLC, these reports include data on the total number of deficiencies identified and the categories in which the identified deficiencies fall. VA headquarters officials expect that these quarterly reports will facilitate the identification of national areas for improvement as well as help them review CLCs' performance on the LTCI reviews over time.

VA Headquarters Cannot Provide Reasonable Assurance That All Deficiencies Are Resolved Because of Weaknesses in Its Process for Responding to Deficiencies

When responding to LTCI-identified deficiencies, VA headquarters does not always maintain clear and complete documentation of the feedback it provides to CLCs regarding their corrective action plans. In addition, VA headquarters does not require VA networks to report on the status of CLCs' implementation of their corrective action plans or to verify CLCs' self-reported compliance with the requirements of the national training and education initiative. Without the ability to determine whether CLCs appropriately responded to feedback, fully implemented their corrective action plans from the 2007 and 2008 LTCI reviews, or fully complied with requirements of the national training and education initiative, and without the ability to determine the status of corrective action plans that CLCs are implementing during LTCI's 2010 and 2011 reviews, VA headquarters does not have reasonable assurance that LTCI-identified deficiencies are resolved.

Lack of clear and complete documentation of feedback. VA headquarters does not always maintain clear and complete documentation of the feedback it provides CLCs about their corrective action plans, which is not consistent with good management practices as outlined in federal internal control standards. According to these standards, internal control activities, such as VA headquarters' feedback, should be clearly and completely documented in a manner that is accurate, timely, and helps provide reasonable assurance that program objectives are being achieved.[28] VA headquarters uses an unsystematic approach for documenting the feedback it provides to CLCs regarding their corrective action plans. The approach relies solely on hard copies of CLCs' action plans that have hand-written notes on them, which are not shared with the VA networks and CLCs, to document the feedback provided during VA headquarters' telephone calls with CLCs. We found that this approach did not always result in clear—that is, understandable to anyone not involved in the telephone feedback calls—and complete documentation. In particular, the documentation we reviewed did not always clearly and completely indicate the specific feedback provided to CLCs, including actions VA headquarters advised CLCs to take to address weaknesses with their corrective action plans. For example, for one CLC we obtained two corrective action plans from VA headquarters. One was an older action plan and the other was a revised action plan. The older action plan contained no notes or any indication of the content of VA headquarters' feedback that resulted in the revised action plan, so we were unable to independently determine whether the revised action plan addressed VA headquarters' feedback. In addition, we found that the plans for 19 of the 50 2007 and 2008 CLC corrective action plans that we reviewed—or about 38 percent of the plans—lacked any notes documenting the feedback that VA headquarters gave CLCs on the telephone calls.

Lack of reporting requirement for VA networks. VA headquarters does not require its networks to report on the status of CLCs' implementation of their corrective action plans, and VA headquarters does not routinely schedule additional telephone calls with CLCs following the submission of initial corrective action plans and VA's initial telephone calls. For example, VA headquarters held additional telephone calls with only 25 percent of CLCs following the 2007 and 2008 LTCI reviews, and 15 percent of the CLCs following the 2010 and 2011 LTCI reviews, as of March 31, 2011. Therefore, VA headquarters does not know whether CLCs fully implemented their plans and corrected all LTCI-identified deficiencies. Federal standards for internal control state that the findings of reviews should be promptly resolved and that information on the status of the findings should be communicated to management so that management can provide reasonable assurance that a program is achieving its objectives—in this case, that CLCs are providing quality care and maintaining veterans' quality of life.[29] VA headquarters officials told us that beyond the initial telephone calls with CLCs, VA headquarters does not receive any additional information from CLCs regarding the implementation status of their corrective action plans. Rather, VA headquarters officials expect the findings of the 2010 and 2011 LTCI reviews will help them determine whether CLCs resolved all deficiencies identified by LTCI in 2007 and 2008—2 or 3 years after the deficiencies were first identified.

Lack of verification requirement for national initiative. We found that VA headquarters relied on self-reported information from CLCs regarding (1) compliance with all four requirements for each of the eight clinical high-risk categories and (2) the percentage of staff that were observed to be proficient in treatments and procedures associated with the categories. VA headquarters did not specify to its networks that they should verify the accuracy of CLCs' self-reported information. Reliance on self-reported information is inconsistent with federal standards for internal control specifying that management should be able to provide reasonable assurance about the accuracy of data—in this case, that VA networks verify the accuracy of CLCs' self-reported information.[30] Although we cannot generalize to all networks, neither of the two VA networks we visited requested documentation to verify CLCs' self-reported information for the national training and education initiative. Further, the 2010 and 2011 LTCI reviews indicate that some CLCs are not in compliance with the requirements for the eight clinical high-risk categories stemming from the 2007 and 2008 reviews. For example, a CLC reported to VA headquarters that by June 2009 it would have a policy in place for training and educating its staff on PICC lines—one of the eight clinical high-risk categories. However, when LTCI reviewed this CLC in 2010, it found that this CLC had failed to provide proper care and treatment when administering medication to a resident through a PICC line. When LTCI asked to see the CLC's policy related to PICC lines, the CLC's staff stated that the CLC did not have one.

VA Headquarters Receives Information about CLCs from Multiple Sources, but Does Not Analyze It to Assess and Manage Risks

In addition to LTCI reviews, VA headquarters obtains information about CLCs from a variety of other sources that could be used to more comprehensively identify risks associated with the care and quality of life of CLC residents. VA headquarters does not analyze all of these sources, and for those sources it does analyze, VA evaluates each source in isolation without comparing the information it receives across all available sources to identify major or commonly cited risks and trends. As a result, VA headquarters' current approach to identifying risks in CLCs may result in missed opportunities to detect patterns and trends in information about the quality of care and quality of life within a CLC or across many CLCs. Without considering information from all available sources and comparing it across different sources, VA headquarters cannot adequately identify and manage risks in CLCs.

VA Headquarters Receives Useful Information about CLCs from Multiple Sources

We found that VA headquarters receives information about the quality of care and quality of life in CLCs from at least nine different sources. The type of information VA headquarters receives from each of these sources, and how often the agency receives it, varies. The nine sources of information about CLCs are the following:

- *LTCI.* Conducts annual unannounced reviews that assess the extent to which CLCs follow 176 federal long-term care standards.[31] LTCI review teams observe the delivery of care for a sample of residents in order to examine such areas as medication management, infection control practices, and respect for residents' rights and dignity. LTCI provides VA headquarters a report of all deficiencies identified. VA headquarters then shares the report with the network and the reviewed CLC. The CLC is expected to correct identified deficiencies.
- *The Joint Commission.* Performs accreditation surveys every 3 years, on average, assessing CLCs' compliance with 227 long-term care standards, such as infection control practices and resident assessments. When The Joint Commission surveyors find noncompliance, they determine whether a systemic problem exists by assessing the CLC's established policies and processes. This determination is the basis for whether CLCs are found deficient in a long-term care standard. VA networks and CLCs receive survey reports from The Joint Commission, which identify specific deficiencies. CLCs are required to resolve the deficiencies within certain time frames in order to maintain accreditation.[32]
- *OIG.* Performs its Combined Assessment Program reviews at VAMCs, including CLCs, about every 3 years. Under this program, OIG reviews selected VAMC activities, including CLC activities, to assess the effectiveness of patient care administration (the process of planning and delivering patient care) and quality management (the process of monitoring quality of care to identify and correct harmful and potentially harmful practices and conditions).[33] CLCs typically are part of each Combined Assessment Program review. Upon completion of each review, OIG issues a report to VA headquarters, the network, and the VAMC, which identifies the VAMC's deficiencies, including any deficiencies identified in the CLC. VA requires VAMCs, including CLCs, to fully resolve deficiencies within a year of the completion of a Combined Assessment Program review.
- *VA Office of the Medical Inspector (OMI).* Conducts investigations to determine the validity of allegations made by complainants regarding the care provided to veterans, including residents of CLCs.[34] If an allegation is validated, the VAMC, including the CLC, is required to address any recommendations made by OMI.[35]

- *System-wide Ongoing Assessment and Review Strategy (SOARS).* Performs reviews of VAMCs, including CLCs, every 3 years to evaluate readiness for some external and internal reviews, such as those by The Joint Commission and OIG.[36] It is a consultative program within VA designed to identify programmatic weaknesses in VAMCs, including CLCs. SOARS teams issue reports to VA networks and VAMCs, including CLCs, with recommendations based on identified deficiencies, and VAMCs and CLCs are expected to implement the recommendations.
- *Quality Measures and Quality Indicators.* Report the percentage of residents in a CLC who have certain conditions, such as a pressure ulcer, or residents who are at risk for developing certain conditions, such as CLC residents who have limited mobility and are at risk of developing a pressure ulcer. CLCs periodically assess residents and enter information about their conditions into a database, which automatically calculates percentage scores for 24 categories of quality measures and quality indicators. Data are available on an ongoing basis.
- *Artifacts of Culture Change Tool.*[37] Reports the extent to which CLCs provided resident-centered care. Using a standard self-assessment tool, CLCs score their own performance in certain areas, such as allowing residents to choose when they eat meals, bathe, and sleep. CLCs report their scores to VA headquarters every 6 months.
- *Issue Briefs.* Provide specific information to VA headquarters officials regarding unusual incidents, such as deaths, disasters, or anything else that happens at a VAMC, including a CLC, that might generate media interest or affect care.[38]
- *Complaints.* Provide information from veterans or their representatives about the quality of care or the quality of life in VAMCs, including CLCs.[39]

VA Headquarters Does Not Consider the Potential Usefulness of All Available Information to Assess and Manage Risks in CLCs

VA headquarters' approach for identifying risks associated with the quality of care and quality of life of CLC residents is deficient in two respects—it does not comprehensively analyze information from all available sources, and it does not compare findings across these sources. Without analyzing information from all available sources and comparing the results, VA headquarters' assessments of risks in CLCs are incomplete. According to federal internal control standards, management should assess the risks the agency may face from both external and internal sources. The standards state that a risk management process includes (1) comprehensively identifying risks associated with achieving an agency's goals (for example, providing quality of care and quality of life in CLCs); (2) estimating the significance of the risks; and (3) determining actions to mitigate the risks, such as developing or clarifying policies or targeting reviews of noncompliant CLCs.[40]

VA Headquarters Does Not Analyze Information from All Available Sources

VA headquarters' current approach relies significantly on the analysis of findings from LTCI reviews of CLCs. VA headquarters also relies on analysis of the findings from The Joint Commission accreditation surveys and the Artifacts of Culture Change tool. (See app. I for a detailed description of these analyses.) While these three separate analyses enable VA headquarters to identify trends in each source of information, such as the most frequently cited deficiencies across all CLCs or the average number of deficiencies per CLC, they do not provide a complete assessment of the risks that would be identified by evaluating all nine sources. Information VA headquarters receives about the quality of care and the quality of life in CLCs from the remaining six sources—OIG, OMI, SOARS, quality measures and quality indicators, issue briefs, and complaints—could also be valuable in identifying patterns in CLC-related findings. VA headquarters officials we interviewed said they do not typically analyze information they receive about CLCs from these six sources because they do not always believe that doing so would be valuable for identifying trends and patterns regarding the quality of care and quality of life in CLCs. For example, VA headquarters officials said that they do not extract CLC-related findings from OIG Combined Assessment Program reviews because the reviews typically do not include enough CLC-related findings to warrant analysis. However, when we analyzed findings from the 77 OIG Combined Assessment Program reviews that were completed at VAMCs that have CLCs between October 1, 2009, and June 20, 2011, we found that 49 of the reviews—or about 64 percent—included at least one finding related to the quality of care or quality of life in a CLC. Without analyzing information from all available sources about the quality of care and quality of life in CLCs, VA headquarters' assessments of risks in CLCs are incomplete.

VA Headquarters Does Not Compare Information across All Available Sources

VA headquarters does not compare information across all sources to identify patterns of findings for an individual CLC, CLCs within a network, or all CLCs nationwide. Rather, VA headquarters analyzes the findings from three sources separately to identify trends in the findings. However, it does not compare the findings from one source to the findings from the other sources. One source's findings, in isolation, may not present the significance of certain risks, especially those that may suggest immediate risks for residents within a given CLC or across all CLCs. However, if related information that VA headquarters receives was compared across different sources concurrently, VA headquarters officials would be better positioned to recognize the risks to CLC residents.

One example we identified of the benefit from considering the usefulness of multiple information sources is in the area of pain management. In this regard, we found that in fiscal years 2009 and 2010, VA headquarters' quality indicator and quality measure data showed that about 25 percent of all long-stay CLC residents and 40 percent of all short-stay CLC residents experienced moderate to severe pain. In June 2007, OMI investigated allegations about the quality of care for a resident at one CLC and found, among other things, that the CLC had failed to adequately manage the resident's pain. Three months later, in September 2007, LTCI conducted a review of the same CLC and found that staff were not performing assessments after administering pain medications to determine whether the medication had been effective. In November 2009, the OIG visited the same CLC as part of a Combined Assessment Program review and found that staff had not documented pain medication effectiveness within the required time frames nearly two-thirds of the time that pain medications were administered. If VA had comprehensively analyzed OMI information—which it does not analyze—along with LTCI information that was available in 2007 and compared this information with the information from the 2009 OIG review and quality indicator and quality measure data, VA headquarters would have been better informed about the significance of the risks and what actions might have helped to mitigate the risks of pain medication management problems at this CLC.

CONCLUSIONS

The 46,000 elderly and disabled veterans annually who are residents in VA's CLCs depend on VA to provide them with quality care and maintain their quality of life. The weaknesses in VA headquarters' process for resolving LTCI-identified deficiencies put veterans at risk of persistent deficiencies that could become more serious over time. VA headquarters officials told us that they intend to use the findings of the 2010 and 2011 LTCI reviews to determine whether deficiencies that were first identified by LTCI 2 to 3 years earlier have been resolved. However, VA headquarters cannot provide reasonable assurance of resolution of deficiencies because it does not (1) clearly document the feedback that it provides to CLCs about corrective action plans for LTCI-identified deficiencies, (2) require VA networks to report on the status of CLCs' implementation of action plans, and (3) verify CLCs' self-reported information about their implementation of the requirements of the national training and education initiative. Unaddressed, these weaknesses in VA headquarters' process for responding to LTCI-identified deficiencies may compromise the quality of care and quality of life of veterans in CLCs.

Even though VA headquarters receives information about the quality of care and quality of life in CLCs from LTCI and a variety of other sources, the agency does not comprehensively analyze all available information to identify and manage risks in CLCs. Because VA headquarters does not analyze information from all available sources, it may be missing opportunities to detect trends and patterns in findings from different information sources for a CLC, CLCs within a network, or all CLCs. Without comprehensively analyzing information from all available sources, VA headquarters cannot fully identify risks in CLCs, estimate the significance of the risks, or take actions to mitigate them.

RECOMMENDATIONS FOR EXECUTIVE ACTION

To provide reasonable assurance that LTCI-identified deficiencies are resolved and that veterans receive quality care and maintain their quality of life in VA CLCs, we recommend that the Secretary of Veterans Affairs direct the Under Secretary for Health to take the following two actions:

- For reviews conducted by LTCI under the current contract and any similar future contracts, (1) clearly and completely document the feedback provided to CLCs about their corrective action plans, (2) require VA networks to provide periodic reports on the status of CLCs' implementation of their corrective action plans, and (3) develop and implement a process for verifying any information reported directly to VA headquarters by CLCs.

- Develop and implement a process to comprehensively identify, estimate, and mitigate risks in CLCs by analyzing and comparing all available information regarding the quality of care and quality of life in CLCs.

AGENCY COMMENTS AND OUR EVALUATION

In its comments on a draft of this report, VA concurred with our recommendations and described the department's planned actions to implement them. VA did not provide technical comments on the draft report.

To address our recommendation that, for reviews conducted by LTCI, VA headquarters should document the feedback provided to CLCs about their corrective action plans, require VA networks to report periodically on the status of CLCs' implementation of corrective action plans, and implement a process for verifying information CLCs report directly to VA headquarters, VA stated that it plans to develop and implement a national feedback process by the end of the second quarter of fiscal year 2012 as part of its response to results from the LTCI reviews. VA stated that the process will include having VA networks work with VAMC leadership to develop a comprehensive action plan to address areas of concern highlighted in the LTCI reviews, using a standardized template for CLCs' corrective action plans, and requiring VAMCs to post corrective action plans on a secure database and provide updated corrective action plans at least monthly. VA indicated that the process will provide access to the status of action plans at any time and that officials from VA headquarters will provide oversight to ensure completion of action plans, including requiring VA networks to validate completion of all action items. VA, however, did not specify in its comments whether its process would include a step to document the feedback provided to CLCs about their corrective actions plans. We believe it is important for VA to document feedback provided to CLCs as part of its process

To address our recommendation that VA headquarters develop and implement a process to comprehensively identify, estimate, and mitigate risks in CLCs by analyzing and comparing all available information regarding quality of care and quality of life, VA stated that it plans to design a process that will use all available information about the quality of care and quality of life in CLCs. VA indicated that this process would allow officials to analyze and compare information for individual CLCs, for CLCs within a VA network, and across all CLCs nationwide. VA intends to design this process during the first quarter of fiscal year 2012 and plans to use the process to analyze and compare CLC information and begin reporting it during the second quarter of fiscal year 2012. We commend this effort and encourage VA to proceed with these plans.

Sincerely yours,

Randall B. Williamson
Director, Health Care

Appendix I. VA Headquarters' Analysis of Information about the Quality of Life and Care in Community Living Centers

Source of information	Frequency of analysis	Description of VA headquarters analysis
Long Term Care Institute, Inc.	Quarterly, annually	• Identify the most frequently cited deficiencies nationally. • Identify the total number of deficiencies per community living center (CLC). • Classify deficiencies identified in each CLC into 1 of 17 different groups (e.g., activities, environment, infection control, medication, etc.). Use these groups to track trends in deficiencies by VA network and by CLC. • Determine whether each CLC was substantially compliant with federal long-term care standards.
The Joint Commission	Annually	• Identify most frequently cited findings for two areas:[a] 1. Direct impact: includes findings that are likely to present an immediate risk to residents' safety or quality of care; for example, resident assessment and pain management. 2. Indirect impact: includes findings that pose less immediate risk to residents' safety or quality of life, but could become more serious over time; for example, care planning and ensuring that corridors, hallways, and doors remain free from obstructions that would prevent exit in the event of a fire. • Calculate average number of findings per CLC.
Quality measures and quality indicators	Quarterly, annually	• Calculate average performance on 30 measures and indicators, by VA network and nationally; for example, percentage of long-stay residents who have experienced moderate to severe pain.
Artifacts of culture change tool	Every 6 months	• Calculate average scores, by VA network and nationally, for areas such as care practices (e.g., allowing residents to choose when they eat, bathe, and sleep) and leadership (e.g., holding regular community meetings that encourage the participation of staff, residents, and families).

Source: GAO analysis of VA data.

[a] In its surveys, The Joint Commission determines whether findings have a direct or an indirect impact on resident care.

End Notes

[1] The remaining $1.2 billion spent for nursing home care was for care provided to veterans in state veterans homes ($652 million) and community nursing homes ($550 million).

[2] VA's model of care for CLC residents emphasizes the delivery of quality health care and the maintenance of a quality of life for CLC residents. Practices that contribute to residents' quality of life include the extent to which CLC staff treat residents with respect and dignity and the extent to which residents are permitted to exercise personal preferences in areas such as the activities they choose to engage in and the food they choose

to eat. See Veterans Health Administration Handbook 1142.01, *Criteria and Standards for VA Community Living Centers* (Aug. 13, 2008).

[3] LTCI is a not-for-profit organization that surveys nursing homes and other residential settings to improve care for residents.

[4] VA had no in-depth reviews of CLCs conducted between October 2008 and September 2010.

[5] The 50 corrective action plans we reviewed were submitted by CLCs that were reviewed by LTCI in 2007 or 2008 and again between September 1, 2010, and March 31, 2011. We chose March 31, 2011, as the final date for inclusion in our sample of 2010 and 2011 LTCI reviews and corrective action plans because VA headquarters requires that LTCI provide a final report 10 days after the completion of an LTCI review. VA headquarters then transmits the review to the CLC, which has up to 30 days to submit its corrective action plan to VA headquarters. Given the time frames within which we could reasonably expect to receive copies of the 2010 and 2011 LTCI reviews and action plans from VA headquarters, we chose to limit the scope of our sample to LTCI reviews that were completed before March 31, 2011.

[6] The corrective action plans and related documentation of the 23 CLCs represent all of the 2010 and 2011 action plans that were available as of March 22, 2011. These 23 CLCs represent about 34 percent of the CLCs included in our sample of LTCI reviews that were completed, as of March 31, 2011. Findings from our review of the sample of 2007 and 2008 corrective action plans, along with findings from our review of the sample of 2010 and 2011 LTCI reviews and corrective action plans, cannot be generalized to all CLCs.

[7] In this report, we use Geriatrics and Extended Care when referring to the Office of Geriatrics and Extended Care.

[8] We selected the VA Mid-Atlantic Health Care Network because it had a high average number of deficiencies per CLC. We selected the VA Northwest Health Network because it had a medium average number of deficiencies per CLC.

[9] GAO, *Standards for Internal Control in the Federal Government*, GAO/AIMD-00-21.3.1 (Washington, D.C.: November 1999).

[10] VA nursing home care is provided in three settings: VA-operated CLCs, community nursing homes, and state veterans homes.

[11] 38 U.S.C. § 1710A(a). These requirements will terminate on December 31, 2013. 38 U.S.C. § 1710A(d). The statute states that these requirements may not be construed as authorizing or requiring that a veteran who was receiving nursing home care in a department nursing home on November 30, 1999, be displaced, transferred, or discharged from the facility. 38 U.S.C. § 1710A(b)(2). Requirements for the provision of nursing home care, like those related to hospital and medical care, are effective in any fiscal year only to the extent and in the amount provided in advance in appropriations acts for such purposes. 38 U.S.C. § 1710(a)(4).

[12] 38 U.S.C. § 1710(a)(2), (3).

[13] In August 2011, VA exercised its option for a second year for reviews to be conducted from September 2011 through August 2012. The cost of the contract for the base year was $3.5 million. If VA exercises all of the options through 2015, the total cost of the contract for 5 years will be $18.3 million.

[14] See Veterans Health Administration Handbook 1100.16, *Accreditation of Veterans Health Administration Medical Facility and Ambulatory Programs* (Sept. 22, 2009). The Joint Commission is an independent organization that accredits and certifies health care organizations and programs in the United States.

[15] Community nursing homes that receive Medicare or Medicaid payments must be inspected by state agencies that contract with the Centers for Medicare & Medicaid Services not later than 15 months after the date of the previous inspection, and the statewide average for inspection of nursing homes must not exceed 12 months. See 42 U.S.C. §§ 1395i-3(g)(2)(A)(iii), 1396r(g)(2)(A)(iii). Community nursing homes are evaluated on compliance with federal long-term care standards, which are codified at 42 C.F.R. Part 483, Subpart B. Community nursing homes may separately contract with The Joint Commission to receive accreditation, although this is not a requirement for receiving Medicare or Medicaid payment.

[16] See Veterans Health Administration Handbook 1142.01, Criteria and Standards for *VA Community Living Centers* (Aug. 13, 2008).

[17] The 29 CLCs that participated in more than one telephone call with VA headquarters after their 2007 or 2008 review were located in 16 of VA's 21 networks.

[18] For immediate jeopardy level findings, LTCI surveyors are required to remain at the CLC until the deficiencies are abated.

[19] To be consistent with criteria used by VA in requiring notification of immediate jeopardy and actual harm deficiencies, our analysis did not include deficiencies classified as isolated actual harm. According to a VA headquarters official, deficiencies classified as isolated actual harm were not included in the criteria due to their limited scope.

[20] A central line is a small tube that is placed in a large vein in the neck, chest, groin, or arm to give fluids, blood, or medications or to do medical tests quickly. A central line can remain for weeks or months, and some patients receive treatment through the line several times a day. A PICC line is a specific type of central line that is placed into a vein in the arm.

[21] The Office of Nursing Services is responsible for devising policies on all issues related to nursing practice and nursing workforce for VA's clinical programs, including nurses in CLCs.

[22] Nutrition and Food Services is responsible for providing overall policy, guidelines, and program development relevant to each health care system and medical center's nutrition and food services.

[23] The Infectious Diseases Program Office is responsible for assisting and developing policy, guidelines, and program development for infectious diseases clinical programs, infection prevention and control, and the infectious diseases health science policy and epidemiology program.

[24] For example, the procedures adopted could include those in the Lippincott Manual of Nursing Practice, which is a manual that outlines clinical guidelines and procedures for nursing practice.

[25] In 2009, VA headquarters specified these requirements in three memorandums from VA's Deputy Under Secretary for Health for Operations and Management. The memorandums were dated January 28, 2009; April 23, 2009; and October 15, 2009. VA required CLCs to submit these eight checklists during calendar years 2009 and 2010.

[26] The requirements for the national training and education initiative were applicable to all 132 CLCs, including the 16 CLCs that LTCI did not review in 2007 and 2008.

[27] The corrective action plans for the clinical high-risk categories were separate from the corrective action plans that all CLCs had to submit directly in response to the LTCI- identified deficiencies.

[28] Control activities are the policies, procedures, techniques, and mechanisms that help ensure that an agency's directives are carried out and that the agency accomplishes its objectives. See GAO/AIMD-00-21.3.1.

[29] See GAO/AIMD-00-21.3.1.

[30] See GAO/AIMD-00-21.3.1.

[31] These are the same long-term care standards used by the Centers for Medicare & Medicaid Services for certifying community nursing homes for participation in the Medicare and Medicaid programs. See 42 C.F.R. Part 483, Subpart B (2010). Every nursing home receiving Medicare or Medicaid payment must be evaluated on these longterm care standards not later than 15 months after the date of the previous evaluation, and the statewide average for these evaluations must not exceed 12 months. See 42 U.S.C. §§ 1395i-3(g)(2)(A)(iii), 1396r(g)(2)(A)(iii).

[32] The Joint Commission has established timelines based on whether a deficiency is considered directly or indirectly related to patient care. Deficiencies directly related to patient care must be resolved within 45 days. Deficiencies indirectly related to patient care must be resolved within 60 days.

[33] The activities selected as topics of the Combined Assessment Program reviews change every 6 to 12 months. According to OIG officials, the selection of activities is based on various internal and external factors: (1) past experience of Combined Assessment Program review team members, (2) trends identified from the OIG complaint system, and (3) problems identified in the private sector (e.g., past concerns regarding the availability of flu vaccines).

[34] Between November 2007 and June 2011, OMI conducted a total of five investigations concerning incidents in CLCs.

[35] Officials from VA networks and VA headquarters are responsible for ensuring that VAMCs, including CLCs, have adequately addressed recommendations made by OMI.

[36] SOARS identifies 28 areas in which a VAMC may be reviewed based on 100 different VA-defined criteria.

[37] Culture change refers to efforts to transform the culture of nursing home care from a medical model, where care is driven by a medical diagnosis, to a person-centered model, where care is driven by the needs of the individual, as affected by medical conditions. The goals of care are achieved in an environment where the resident is respected, treated with dignity, and invited to be an active participant in the resident's own care. See Veterans Health Administration Handbook 1142.01, *Criteria and Standards for VA Community Living Centers* (Aug. 13, 2008).

[38] Instances that may trigger an issue brief include a homicide or suicide on VA property, significant clinical incidents or outcomes negatively affecting a veteran or group of veterans, or a breach of information security.

[39] These complaints are separate from allegations submitted to OMI.

[40] See GAO/AIMD-00-21.3.1.

In: Veteran Injuries, Disorders and Medical Care Service
Editors: Jessica Michaels and Jesse E. Levine
ISBN: 978-1-62081-302-7

Chapter 8

VETERANS HEALTH ADMINISTRATION: COMMUNITY-BASED OUTPATIENT CLINICS*

Sidath Viranga Panangala and Bryce H. P. Mendez

SUMMARY

In the early 1990s, the Veterans Health Administration (VHA)—one of the three administrations of the Department of Veterans Affairs (VA)—began developing a strategy to expand its capacity to provide outpatient primary care, especially for veterans who had to travel long distances to receive care at VA facilities. To facilitate access to primary care closer to where veterans reside, VHA began implementing a system for approving and establishing Community-Based Outpatient Clinics (CBOCs).

A CBOC is a fixed health care site that is geographically distinct or separate from its parent VA medical facility. A CBOC can be either VA-owned and VA-staffed or contracted to Healthcare Management Organizations (HMO). Regardless of how it is administered, a CBOC must have the necessary professional medical staff, access to diagnostic testing and treatment capability, and the referral arrangements needed to ensure continuity of health care for current or eligible veteran patients. VA policies require all CBOCs to be operated in a manner that provides veterans with consistent, safe, high-quality health care.

CBOCs are managed at the Veterans Integrated Service Network (VISN) level, and planning and development of a new CBOC is based on the VA's need, available resources, local market circumstances, and veteran preference.

In FY2010, VA expects to have a total of 833 operational CBOCs throughout the United States and its territories to serve over 2.8 million veteran patients. In addition to primary care, CBOCs provide mental health services, management of acute and chronic medical conditions, and pharmacy benefits, among other services. It should be noted that the type of medical services available at a CBOC can vary from clinic to clinic.

This report provides an overview of VA's rationale in establishing CBOCs, describes how they are managed and administered, discusses medical services provided at CBOCs, and summarizes what is known about the quality and cost of providing care in CBOCs

---

* This is an edited, reformatted and augmented version of a Congressional Research Service publication, CRS Report *for Congress* R41044, *from* www.crs.gov, *p*repared for Members and Committees of Congress, *dated* January 28, 2010.

compared to primary care clinics at VA Medical Centers. Lastly, it describes the process for developing a new CBOC.

INTRODUCTION

Congress is interested in increasing access to care for veterans closer to where they reside.[1] The establishment of Community-Based Outpatient Clinics (CBOCs) is viewed by some as one method of increasing access to care.[2] This report provides an overview of the impetus for the Department of Veterans Affairs (VA) to establish CBOCs, describes how they are managed and administered, discusses medical services provided at CBOCs, and summarizes what is known about the quality and cost of providing care in CBOCs compared to primary care clinics at Department of Veterans Affairs Medical Centers (VAMCs). Lastly, it describes the process for developing a new CBOC.

The VA Health Care System

The Department of Veterans Affairs provides a range of benefits and services to veterans who meet certain eligibility rules, including hospital and medical care, disability compensation and pensions,[3] education,[4] vocational rehabilitation and employment services, assistance to homeless veterans,[5] home loan guarantees,[6] and administration of life insurance, as well as traumatic injury protection insurance for servicemembers and death benefits that cover burial expenses. VA carries out its programs nationwide through the Veterans Benefits Administration (VBA), Veterans Health Administration (VHA), National Cemetery Administration, and the Board of Veterans Appeals (BVA).

VHA is a direct service provider rather than a health insurer or payer of health care. VA health care services are generally available to all honorably discharged veterans of the U.S. Armed Forces who are enrolled in VA's health care system.[7]

Based on a priority enrollment system, veteran enrollees are placed into priority groups. Under this system, VA decides annually whether its appropriations are adequate to serve all enrolled veterans. If not, VA may stop enrolling those in the lowest-priority groups.[8]

The VA's health care system is organized into 21 geographically defined Veterans Integrated Service Networks (VISNs). In FY2009, VHA operated an estimated 153 medical centers, 135 nursing homes, 783 ambulatory care and community-based outpatient clinics (CBOCs), 6 independent outpatient clinics, and 271 Readjustment Counseling Centers (Vet Centers).[9] VHA also operates 10 mobile outpatient clinics.

The VHA pays for care provided to veterans by private-sector providers on a fee basis under certain circumstances. Inpatient and outpatient care are also provided in the private sector to eligible dependents of veterans under the Civilian Health and Medical Program of the Department of Veterans Affairs (CHAMPVA).

The VHA also provides grants for construction of state-owned nursing homes and domiciliary facilities and collaborates with the Department of Defense (DOD) in sharing health care resources and services.

Apart from providing direct patient care to veterans, VHA's other statutory missions are to conduct medical research, to serve as a contingency back up to the Department of Defense

(DOD) medical system during a national security emergency, to provide support to the National Disaster Medical System and the Department of Health and Human Services as necessary, and to train health care professionals in order to provide an adequate supply of health personnel for VA and the Nation.

The next section provides a brief overview on the rationale for establishing CBOCs.

TRANSFORMATION OF VHA AND ESTABLISHMENT OF CBOCS

Since the early 1920s, the VA health care system had been primarily a hospital-based inpatient health care system.[10] Beginning with the 1960s, Congress gradually expanded eligibility for outpatient care.[11] Several research studies reported that a "large proportion of VA hospital admissions in the mid 1980s and early 1990s were non-acute and could have been treated in an outpatient setting if ambulatory care services had been available geographically."[12] Another study found that the "lack of geographic access to VA outpatient care can lead to higher risk of readmission post-discharge."[13]

In the mid-1990s VA recognized that its system might want to respond to certain changes taking place in the private health care market and began a process of restructuring its health care delivery network. VA established regional networks (Veterans Integrated Service Networks [VISNs]) and decentralized certain budgetary authorities to these networks.[14] Furthermore, advances in medical technology, such as laser and other minimally invasive surgical techniques, allowed care previously provided in hospitals to be provided on an outpatient basis. VA also began developing a strategy to expand its capacity to provide outpatient primary care, especially for veterans who had to travel long distances to receive care at VA facilities.[15] To facilitate access to primary care closer to where veterans reside, VHA began implementing a system for approving and establishing CBOCs.[16] In January 1994, the VHA hospital in Amarillo, TX—now located in Childress, TX—established what is generally recognized as the first VHA community based clinic.[17] Prior to the establishment of this clinic, to establish a CBOC, a clinic had to have a workload of 3,000 visits or more and had to be located at least 100 miles or three hours travel time away from the nearest VHA hospital. In 1995, VHA issued a directive to eliminate these restrictions and to expand its network of CBOCs.[18] New CBOC planning criteria were based on, among other things, (1) eligible veteran population, (2) services to be provided, (3) costs of available alternatives, and (4) sources of funds.[19] The current process of developing CBOCs is discussed later in this report.

Since VHA initiated its CBOC initiative in 1995, over 700 clinics have opened.[20] *Figure 1* displays the number of active CBOCs for each fiscal year from 1999 through projected 2010.

Generally a CBOC is defined as a fixed health care site that is geographically distinct or separate from its parent medical facility.[21] This site can be VA-operated, contracted, or a combination of the two; however, CBOCs are required to have the necessary professional medical staff, access to diagnostic testing and treatment capability, and referral arrangements to ensure the continuity of care for current and eligible veteran patients. A CBOC can provide primary care, specialty care, subspecialty care, mental health, and pharmacy benefits. It should be noted that services can vary from clinic to clinic.

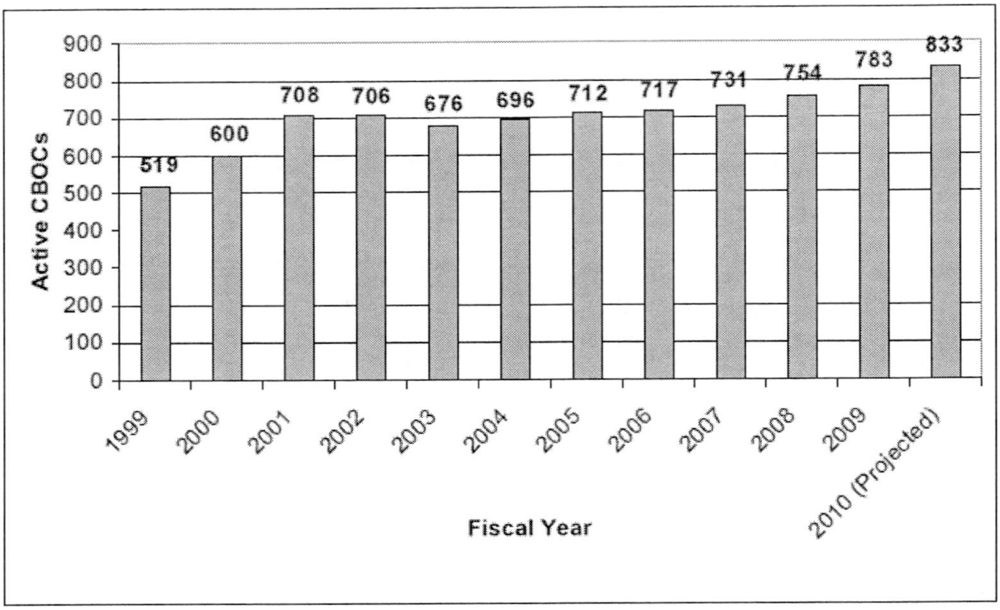

Source: Chart adapted by Congressional Research Service, from Department of Veterans Affairs, Office of Inspector General, Informational Report, Community-Based Outpatient Clinic Cyclical Reports, Report No. 08-00623-169, Washington, DC, July 16, 2009, p. 3. Data for FY2009 adapted from Department of Veterans Affairs, Veterans Health Administration, Office of Legislative Programs, December 2009. Data for FY2010 are adapted from the Department of Veterans Affairs, FY2010 Budget Submission: Medical Programs and Information Technology Programs, Volume 2, Washington, DC, May 2009, pp. 1E-4.

Notes: In some years, services In some CBOCs are suspended and transferred to nearby CBOCs, hence the decline in active CBOCs in those years. Based on the FY2010 Budget Submission, VA expects to open 50 additional CBOCs in FY2010.

Figure 1. Active Community-Based Outpatient Clinics, FY1999-FY2010.

Generally a CBOC is defined as a fixed health care site that is geographically distinct or separate from its parent medical facility.[21] This site can be VA-operated, contracted, or a combination of the two; however, CBOCs are required to have the necessary professional medical staff, access to diagnostic testing and treatment capability, and referral arrangements to ensure the continuity of care for current and eligible veteran patients. A CBOC can provide primary care, specialty care, subspecialty care, mental health, and pharmacy benefits. It should be noted that services can vary from clinic to clinic.

There are currently 783 active CBOCs throughout the United States and its territories, including American Samoa, Guam, Puerto Rico, and the Virgin Islands.

Over 2.8 million patients were seen at CBOCs during FY2008.[22] According to various studies conducted by the VA, CBOCs have been able to serve veterans in a more efficient and effective manner by improving access to health care services and providing high quality primary and mental health care.[23] The next section discusses how CBOCs are managed throughout the VA health care system.

Administration and Management of CBOCs

All Community-Based Outpatient Clinics operate under the supervision and guidance of a single VA hospital or medical center (VAMC). The parent VAMC maintains administrative responsibility for its CBOC(s), specifically with respect to maintaining quality of care (discussed later in this report).

CBOCs are operated by VA and/or contracted staff. In general, CBOCs fall into three major categories:[24]

- VA-Owned—a CBOC that is owned and staffed by VA personnel. The facility space is also owned by VA.
- Leased—a CBOC where the space is leased (contracted) but staffed by VA personnel.
- Contracted—a CBOC where the space and the staff are not VA personnel. This is typically a Healthcare Management Organization (HMO) type provider where there can be multiple sites associated with a single station identifier.

Table 1 displays the number and percent distribution of CBOCs by these three categories for FY2009.

Table 1. CBOCs by Category, FY2009

Type of CBOC	Number of CBOCs	Percentage
VA-Owned	84	10.7
Leased	497	63.5
Contracted	202	25.8
Total	783	100.0

Source: Department of Veterans Affairs, Veterans Health Administration, Office of Legislative Affairs, December 2009.

Notes: Data are current as of September 30, 2009. For FY2009, VA reported having an estimated total of 803 CBOCs in Department of Veterans Affairs, FY2010 Budget Submission: Medical Programs and Information Technology Programs, Vol.2, Washington, DC, May 2009, pp. 1E-4. CRS has been unable to reconcile this discrepancy.

Contracts for CBOCs

The Veterans' Health Care Eligibility Reform Act (P.L. 104-262) authorized VA to obtain health care resources by entering into contracts or other agreements with any health care facility, entity, or individual. There are three statutes in current law that authorize the VA to enter into contracts for establishing CBOCs:

- Title 38 United States Code (U.S.C.) §8153—allows the VA to obtain health care resources such as health care providers, other entities or individuals. Contracts may be used to obtain professional services alone or a comprehensive practice to include the physical plant where the services are provided.

- Title 38 U.S.C. §7409—authorizes the VA to enter into contracts with schools of medicine, dentistry, podiatry, optometry and nursing. Also included in this statute are clinics and other groups or individuals capable of providing medical specialist service to VA facilities.
- Title 38 U.S.C. §8111—authorizes the VA to enter into agreements with the Department of Defense (DOD) to share health care resources. This statute may be used to establish CBOCs at DOD facilities using DOD personnel, VA personnel, or a combination of DOD and VA personnel.

For contracted CBOCs, the contractor is required to provide health care staff, medical facilities, medical equipment, supplies, and all administrative functions sufficient to achieve the contracted level of care in a manner consistent with VHA standards, and meet the requirements and guidelines set forth in the most recent edition of the Joint Commission on the Accreditation of Healthcare Organization (JCAHO, now called The Joint Commission) accreditation manuals. In general, under contracted care the contactor refers veterans to the nearest VAMC for specialty care, extensive diagnostic work, and non-emergency hospitalization. Under the contract, VA requires the contractor to utilize the VA's Computerized Patient Record System (CPRS) for documentation of all patient-related care, including clinical care provided, appointment management, completion of clinical reminders, requests for consultation, scheduling or ordering medications using the VA formulary, requests for prosthetics, and any other computer functions related to patient care. CBOCs are typically open a minimum of five days a week, for a minimum of 40 hours. These days and times could change based on the contract.

When a CBOC contract is up for renewal, it is subject to review by the VA Central Office and approval by the Secretary of Veterans Affairs. In addition to the description of the contract terms, the VISN or facility is required to submit an informational fact sheet to include justification for continued operation of the CBOC under a contract versus a VA-staffed model, and supporting demographic, utilization, and cost information. Results of this review can indicate either a renewal of the current contract, solicitation of a new contract, or conversion to a VA-staffed model CBOC.

Contract CBOCs (and their providers) operate under a capitated payment system, and the contractor is paid a monthly capitated rate for each enrolled patient.[25] For newly enrolled patients, payments commence with the month in which the patient is first seen. The next section of the report discusses the establishment of CBOCs in collaboration with the Department of Defense (DOD) and the Department of Health and Human Services/Indian Health Services (IHS).

CBOC Collaborations with DOD and HIS

In addition to contracting for CBOC services, the VA has established memorandum of understanding (MOU) agreements with both the Department of Defense (DOD) and Department of Health and Human Services/Indian Health Services (IHS) to establish CBOCs. VA/DOD agreements may come in many forms:[26]

- VA may use DOD space to treat VA patients only.
- DOD may use VA space to treat DOD patients only.
- VA and DOD may use common space, but each treats its own beneficiaries. Ancillary services may be contracted out or provided to both beneficiaries in the joint CBOC.
- VA and DOD may use common space to treat the combined patient populations.

VHA has also entered into sharing agreements with IHS to enhance access to health care services to American Indian and Alaska Native veterans. These agreements tend to offer IHS land or facility space for a VA-staffed CBOC, while allowing IHS providers to utilize the VA's health information technology.[27] According to VA, CBOCs operating under these joint partnerships enable sharing of resources, facilities, and personnel between VA and DOD or IHS to increase access to, and provide, primary, and mental health care.[28]

MEDICAL SERVICES IN CBOCS

In general, all veterans receiving care through VA are provided a standard medical benefits package to include preventive care,[29] inpatient[30] and outpatient[31] diagnostic and treatment services,[32] and medication and medical supplies.[33]

Services delivered to veterans at CBOCs vary, however, primary care and mental health services are generally provided at all CBOCs. Primary care includes, but is not limited to, assessment, diagnosis, and medically necessary treatment(s) for physiological and pathological conditions not requiring referral to specialty care or inpatient hospital services. Care is directed toward health promotion and disease prevention, management of acute and chronic medical conditions, and pharmacological management. Many sites include at least one mental health provider, most of whom are psychologists. [34] Research has indicated that CBOCs have enhanced mental health services through VA-mandated routine screening for depression, problem drinking, traumatic brain injury (TBI), post-traumatic stress disorder (PTSD), and military sexual trauma (MST).[35] Psychiatrists, social workers, and mental health nurses are also utilized and work together with primary care staff to serve the mental health needs of veterans. CBOC patients requiring specialty care, inpatient hospital services, or extended medical services are often referred to the parent VA medical facility.

ACCESS, QUALITY, AND COST OF CARE

There have been several research studies on access, quality of care, and cost of providing care through CBOCs. To study if CBOCs provide consistent, safe, and high-quality care, performance evaluations were initiated in 1998 at the request of the VA Undersecretary of Health. A plan was formulated by the Department's Health Services Research and Development Service to create performance measures to evaluate individual CBOCs and the program as a whole in several domains: access to care, cost, mental health, quality, satisfaction, and utilization.[36] Based on data obtained from three performance reports,[37] several studies on access and utilization, quality of care, patient perceptions of care, and cost of care were published in 2002.[38] These published studies provide some analysis of the quality and cost of care provided through CBOCs.

Access to Care

One research study has indicated that CBOCs have improved geographic access to primary care and mental health services to veterans.[39] According to this study, increases in the number of clinics have improved geographic access for veterans in underserved areas resulting in a substantial increase in the number of veterans from these underserved areas who use VA services. Furthermore, while CBOCs provide closer access points to VA health care services, it may also reduce the need or amount required for beneficiary mileage travel reimbursements.[40]

Ensuring Quality of Care

VA's intent in establishing Community-Based Outpatient Clinics was to increase access to primary care and health services for veterans.[41] Though CBOCs can be located in a variety of geographic areas, ranging from rural to urban, VA policies require that veterans receive a uniform standard of care at all VHA health care facilities to ensure continuity of care and quality for the veteran. For contract CBOCs, services must be comparable to services provided to veterans seen at VA-staffed CBOCs and must adhere to the standards set forth in VA regulations and policies. Generally these standards include, but are not limited to, quality, patient safety, and performance.[42]

With regard to clinical indicators, the Office of Quality and Performance provides annual feedback on CBOC performance, including patient satisfaction surveys, preventive care, and clinical guidelines.[43] In addition to timely administrative and clinical evaluations, all CBOCs are required to be integrated into their parent VAMC quality management program and meet the standards of The Joint Commission. By delegating quality assurance and quality improvement to individual VISNs, VA is able to assess CBOC compliance to evidence-based standards of care and to investigate further if facilities fall short of requirements or expected standards. During the CBOC performance evaluation process, VISNs may decide not to open a planned clinic or to close an operating clinic based on the CBOC's ability to accommodate veterans from the service area at a different community-based site, inability to contract care in the community, and/or inability to acquire adequate staffing or site accommodations.[44]

Systematic reviews on administrative and managerial aspects of CBOCs are also conducted by the VA Office of Inspector General (OIG), as requested by Congress.[45] The results and recommendations made by OIG are intended to ensure that CBOCs are "operated in a manner that provides veterans with consistent, safe, high-quality health care in accordance with VA policies and procedures."[46] Recent CBOC inspections, which have varied between sites, address a variety of areas, including ensuring patients' auditory privacy during check-in, examining CBOC access for disabled patients, measures to secure and protect health records, ensuring clinical competencies, monitoring collaborative practice of physician assistants, ensuring quality and safety standards with dispensing outpatient medications, providing oversight and enforcement in accordance with contract terms and conditions, and improving the physician privileges (and reprivileging) process, among other things.[47]

There have also been some studies done on quality of care delivered at CBOCs. One published study has shown that overall CBOCs are providing a similar level quality of care as primary care clinics at parent VAMCs.[48] According to the authors of this study, when data from the VHAs Prevention Index (PI) and Chronic Disease Care Index (CDCI)[49] were compared for both CBOCs and parent VAMCs, "CBOCs in aggregate were not significantly different from parent VAMCs on 15 of the 16 Prevention Index and Chronic Disease Care Index indicators."[50] The PI and CDCI measure the compliance of VA providers with nationally accepted clinical guidelines for primary prevention, early disease detection of patients with chronic diseases such as diabetes and hypertension.[51] Another study comparing quality of care between contract CBOCs and VA-staffed CBOCs found that based on "two measures—flu shot rate among chronic obstructive pulmonary disease (COPD) patients and retinal exam rate among diabetes patients"—quality was similar in both VA-staffed CBOCs and contract CBOCs.[52]

Cost of Treating Veterans in CBOCs

Comparative cost studies of CBOCs and primary care clinics at VAMCs have focused on costs per patient, costs per visit, and total direct costs. Increased geographic access, costs to the patient in drive time, and increased access to VA health care have also been reviewed.

Table 2. Costs of Patients in CBOCs and Parent VAMC Primary Care Clinics

Cost Variables	CBOC	Parent VAMC Clinics
Direct Cost per Primary Care Visit	$75.65	$77.39
Direct Primary Care Cost per Patient	$172.27	$193.54
Direct Specialty Care Cost per Patient	$209.24	$553.19
Direct Ancillary Cost per Patient	$218.67	$462.52
Direct Inpatient Cost per Patient	$49.89	$344.40
Total Direct Costs per Patient	$650.07	$1,553.65
Sample Size	6,546	101,598

Source: Chart adapted by Congressional Research Service, from Matthew L. Maciejewski, Michael K. Chapko, and Ashley N. Hedeen, et al., "VA Community-Based Outpatient Clinics: Cost Performance Measures," Medical Care, vol. 40, no. 7 (June 2002), p. 591.

Notes: Sample examined includes 18 VA-staffed CBOCS and 14 VA Medical Centers, in which four pair of CBOCs had a common VAMC. Contract CBOCs were not included in this study due to extreme variability in cost estimates and the inability to separate direct and indirect costs.

In general, these studies have found that CBOC costs are lower than costs for patients receiving care at parent VAMC primary care clinics. One specific goal set by VA in transitioning from hospital-based care to outpatient care was to reduce the cost-per-user amount by 30%.[53] In a recent study on the cost comparisons of CBOCs versus parent VAMC clinics, the total direct costs were lower for VA-staffed CBOC patients because of "lower specialty and ancillary care costs."[54]

While this may be attributable to substituting primary care at CBOCs for expensive specialty and ancillary care at VAMCs, according to the authors of this study, this alternative is able to provide care at a lower cost than the traditional delivery model in VA Medical Centers. *Table 2* illustrates the varying costs per patient for patients seen at a CBOC versus a VAMC primary care clinic.

In 2000, a VA performance evaluation of CBOC costs and access found that VA-staffed CBOC patients had higher average direct costs per primary care visit than VAMC patients.[55] This is attributable to a variety of factors, including CBOC providers practicing more resource intensive care, providing a greater range or different set of services to their patients than VAMC providers, and the need for improved access and convenience of primary care. When ancillary costs per patient per visit are included with direct primary care costs, CBOC patients had lower total care costs than those at VAMCs. Lower total direct costs for CBOC patients can be attributable to the physical separation of CBOC primary care and VAMC specialty clinics, additional procedural requirements for specialist referrals, better unmeasured general health, and possibly CBOC patients using non-VA services for a larger portion of their total care.

According to VA, CBOCs may offer a cost-effective alternative to providing primary care at parent VAMC clinics while improving geographic access for veterans. Further study and comparative analysis of cost data would be useful to confirm these results using patient-level data on a larger sample of patients and also including contract CBOCs.[56]

Current Process for Developing a New CBOC

This section discusses the current process for planning and establishing CBOCs. As stated previously, in 1995, VHA reorganized its health care delivery network into 22 geographically defined Veterans Integrated Service Networks (VISN).[57] At the same time, VHA gave VISN Directors the decision-making responsibility to establish CBOCs. However, the Departments of Veterans Affairs and Housing and Urban Development, Independent Agencies Appropriations Act of 1990 (P.L. 101-144), changed this, mandating that VA notify Congress of its intent to open a CBOC no later than 14 days prior to taking irrevocable action.[58]

Planning for a new CBOC is done at the VISN level. This allows VA decisions regarding the need for new CBOCs to be made in the context of available resources, as well as local market circumstances and veteran preferences. Plans for activating CBOCs are included in the VISN's strategic plans and use the most current veteran data, such as number of veterans in the geographic location and potential enrollment figures, among other things. CBOCs are funded primarily through existing VISN resources.

As a result, planning for CBOCs is also dependent on fiscal year budget forecasts and allocations. VISN chief fiscal officers must certify that the facility can maintain services given current budget scenarios at the same time the CBOC business plan is being reviewed against national planning criteria.

Review Process for CBOC Business Plans

The following steps briefly describe the review process of new CBOC business plans:

- VISNs submit CBOC business plans for review against national planning criteria (see below). VISNs submit plans for CBOCs that were (1) identified in the Capital Asset Realignment for Enhanced Services (CARES) plan,[59] or (2) identified in the network strategic plan and/or updates provided to the Deputy Under Secretary for Health for Operations and Management (DUSHOM) on previous plans for CBOC activation. VISNs certify that the CBOC can be implemented within existing funds once approved.
- National review panels (NRP) convene to review proposals against national planning criteria. The national planning criteria include the following: if the CBOC is located in a market not meeting VA access guidelines; if there are space deficits at the parent facility; the number of users and enrollees; market penetration; unique considerations—such as targeted minority veteran populations, geographic barriers, highly rural and/or low population density, medically underserved, DOD sharing opportunities, and parking and transit issues at parent facility; cost effectiveness of proposed sites; impact on specialty care, and waiting times.
- The NRP submits results of the review with recommendations to DUSHOM.
- DUSHOM obtains approvals from Under Secretary for Health and Secretary.
- The Office of Management and Budget (OMB) reviews the CBOC plans.
- VA provides notice to Congress.

Figure 2 provides time frames involved in the CBOC planning and approval process. According to VA, it generally takes about two years from the planning process to the time when patients start receiving treatment.[60]

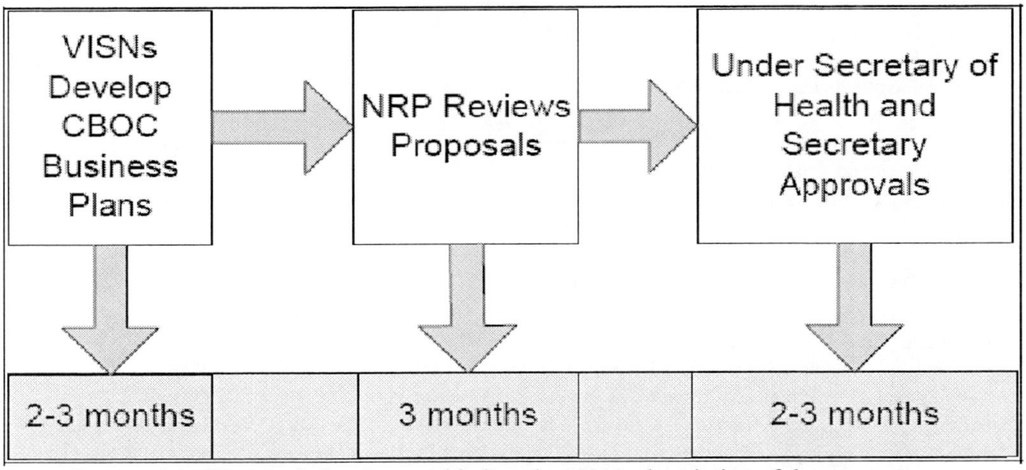

Source: Congressional Research Service graphic based on VA's description of the process.

Notes: VISN = Veterans Integrated Services Network; CBOC = Community-Based Outpatient Clinic; NRP = National Review Panels.

Figure 2. CBOC Planning and Approval Process.

End Notes

[1] U.S. Congress, House Committee on Appropriations, Subcommittee on Military Construction, Veterans Affairs, and Related Agencies, Review of VA Challenges, 111th Cong., 1st sess., March 12, 2009, p. 143.

[2] Ibid. U.S. Congress, House Committee on Appropriations, Consolidated Appropriations Act, 2010, conference report to accompany H.R. 3288 , 111th Cong., 1st sess., December 8, 2009, H.Rept. 111-366 (Washington: GPO, 2009), pp. 1351-1352.

[3] For detailed information on disability compensation and pension programs, see CRS Report RL33323, Veterans Affairs: Benefits for Service-Connected Disabilities, by Douglas Reid Weimer, and CRS Report RS22804, Veterans' Benefits: Pension Benefit Programs, by Christine Scott and Carol D. Davis.

[4] For details on education benefits, see CRS Report R40723, Educational Assistance Programs Administered by the U.S. Department of Veterans Affairs, by Cassandria Dortch.

[5] For detailed information on homeless veterans programs, see CRS Report RL34024, Veterans and Homelessness, by Libby Perl.

[6] For details on the home loan guarantee program see, CRS Report RS20533, VA-Home Loan Guaranty Program: An Overview, by Bruce E. Foote.

[7] For most veterans, entry into the veterans' health care system begins by completing the application for enrollment. Some veterans are exempt from the enrollment requirement if they meet special eligibility requirements. Veterans do not need to apply for enrollment in the VA's health care system if they fall into one of the following categories: veterans with a service-connected disability rated 50% or more (percentage ratings represent the average impairment in earning capacity resulting from disease and injuries encountered as a result of or incident to military service; those with a rating of 50% or more are placed in Priority Group 1); less than one year has passed since the veteran was discharged from military service for a disability that the military determined was incurred or aggravated in the line of duty, but the VA has not yet rated; or the veteran is seeking care from the VA only for a service-connected disability (even if the rating is only 10%). For a description of priority groups see, CRS Report R40737, Veterans Medical Care: FY2010 Appropriations, by Sidath Viranga Panangala.

[8] For more on eligibility for VA Health Care, see CRS Report R40737, Veterans Medical Care: FY2010 Appropriations, by Sidath Viranga Panangala.

[9] Department of Veterans Affairs, FY2010 Budget Submission: Medical Programs and Information Technology Programs, Volume 2, Washington, DC, May 2009, pp. 1E-4. E-mail communication from Department of Veterans Affairs, Veterans Health Administration, Office of Legislative Programs, December 2009.

[10] United States Veterans' Bureau, Annual Report of the Director United States Veterans Bureau for FY1924, December 1, 1924, p. 21.

[11] For a detailed description of the evolution of eligibility for VA health care, see CRS Report RL32961, Veterans' Health Care Issues in the 109th Congress, by Sidath Viranga Panangala.

[12] As cited in John C. Fortney et al., "VA Community-Based Outpatient Clinics: Access and Utilization Performance Measures," Medical Care, vol. 40, no. 7 (July 2002), p. 562.

[13] Ibid.

[14] Kenneth Kizer, John Demakis, and John Feussner, "Reinventing VA health care: Systematizing Quality Improvement and Quality Innovation." Medical Care. vol. 38, no. 6 (June 2000), Suppl 1:I7-16.

[15] U.S. General Accounting Office, VA Community Clinics: Networks' Efforts to Improve Veterans' Access to Primary Care Vary, HEHS-98-116, June 15, 1998, p. 4.

[16] Michael K. Chapko et al., "Evaluation of the Department of Veterans Affairs Community-Based Outpatient Clinics," Medical Care, vol. 40, no. 7 (July 2002), p. 556.

[17] Department of Veterans Affairs, Office of Inspector General, Informational Report, Community-Based Outpatient Clinic Cyclical Reports, Report No. 08-00623-169, Washington, DC, July 16, 2009, p.1.

[18] Department of Veterans Affairs, VHA Directive 10-95-017, Veterans Health Administration Interim Policy for Planning and Activating Department of Veterans Affairs Access Points. February 8, 1995.

[19] Department of Veterans Affairs, Veterans Health Administration, VHA Directive 96-049, Veterans Health Administration Policy For Planning And Activating Community Based Outpatient Clinics, August 7, 1996.

[20] Ibid.

[21] Department of Veterans Affairs, Planning and Activating Community-Based Outpatient Clinics, VHA Handbook: 1006.1, Washington, DC, May 2004.

[22] E-mail communication from Department of Veterans Affairs, Veterans Health Administration, Office of Legislative Programs, December 2009.

[23] John C. Fortney, Matthew L. Maciejewski, and James J. Warren, et al., "Does Improving Geographic Access to VA Primary Care Services Impact Patients' Patterns of Utilization and Costs?" Inquiry, vol. 42 (Spring 2005), pp. 29-42. Robert Rosenheck, "Primary Care Satellite Clinics and Improved Access to General and Mental Health Clinics," Health Services Research, vol. 35, no. 4 (October 2000), pp. 777-790. Ashley N. Hedeen, Patrick J. Heagerty, and John C. Fortney, et al., "VA Community-Based Outpatient Clinics: Quality of Care Performance Measures," Medical Care, vol. 40, no. 7 (July 2002), pp. 570-577. Steven J. Borosky, David B. Nelson, and John C. Fortney, et al., "VA Community-Based Outpatient Clinics: Performance Measures Based on Patient Perceptions of Care," Medical Care, vol. 40, no. 7 (June 2002), pp. 578-586.

[24] Department of Veterans Affairs, Office of Inspector General, Informational Report, Community-Based Outpatient Clinic Cyclical Reports, Report No. 08-00623-169, Washington, DC, July 16, 2009, p. 3.

[25] Capitation payment systems are based on the number of people to be served by the provider. Here, the VA pays a monthly per capita payment to the provider institution to deliver a packet of services to enrolled veterans.

[26] Department of Veterans Affairs, Veterans Health Administration, Guidelines and Templates for Establishing Contracts for Community-Based Outpatient Clinics, Washington, DC, September 20, 2004.

[27] Health information technology includes the VA's electronic medical record system, bar code medication administration and telemedicine. Memorandum of Understanding between the VA/Veterans Health Administration and HHS/Indian Health Service, February 25, 2003.

[28] Congressional Research Service, staff site visit to Alaska VA Health Care System, August 24, 2009.

[29] Preventive care services include immunizations, physical examinations, health care assessments, screening tests, and health education programs.

[30] Inpatient diagnostic and treatment includes emergency inpatient care in VA facilities, medical and surgical procedures, mental health and substance abuse.

[31] Medications and medical supplies include prescription medications, over-the-counter medications and medical and surgical supplies. Prescriptions must generally be from a VA provider and covered under the VA's national formulary system.

[32] Outpatient diagnostic and treatment includes emergency outpatient care in VA facilities, medical and surgical procedures, chiropractic care, mental health, bereavement counseling and substance abuse.

[33] 38 C.F.R. § 17.38.

[34] Antonette M. Zeiss and Bradley E. Karlin, "Integrating Mental Health and Primary Care Services in the Department of Veterans Affairs Health Care System," Journal of Clinical Psychology in Medical Settings, vol. 15, no. 1 (February 2008), p. 73-78.

[35] Ibid.

[36] Department of Veterans Affairs, CBOC Performance Evaluation Project, CBOC Characteristics, Washington, DC, February 17, 1999.

[37] Department of Veterans Affairs, Health Services Research and Development Service, CBOC Performance Evaluation Project, 2000, http://www.research.va.gov/ resources/ pubs /cboc. cfm.

[38] See Medical Care, vol. 40, no. 7 (June 2002), pp. 555-595.

[39] Robert Rosenheck, "Primary Care Satellite Clinics and Improved Access to General and Mental Health Services," Health Services Research, vol. 35, no. 4 (October 2000), pp. 777-790.

[40] Eligible beneficiaries are reimbursed for travel to or from VA facilities or other places for the purposes of examination, treatment or care. For further details on the beneficiary travel program see CRS Report R40737, Veterans Medical Care: FY2010 Appropriations, by Sidath Viranga Panangala.

[41] U.S. Government Accountability Office, VA Health Care: Community-Based Clinics Improve Primary Care, Washington, DC, March 2001.

[42] Department of Veterans Affairs, Informational Report for the Community-Based Outpatient Clinic Cyclical Reports, 08-00623-169, Washington, DC, January 16, 2009.

[43] Department of Veterans Affairs, Veterans Health Administration, Planning and Activating Community-Based Outpatient Clinics, VHA Handbook 1006.1, Washington, DC, May 9, 2004.

[44] Ibid.

[45] A request for the OIG to conduct systematic reviews of CBOCs was made in H.Rept. 110-775 to accompany H.R. 6599, the Military Construction, Veterans Affairs and Related Agencies Appropriation Bill for FY2009.

[46] Department of Veterans Affairs, Office of Inspector General, Health Care Inspection: Community-Based Outpatient Clinic Reviews: Macon and Albany, GA, Beaver Dam, WI, Rockford, IL, Sioux City, IA, Aberdeen, SD, Waterloo, IA and Galesburg, IL, 09-01446-37, Washington, DC, December 2, 2009.

[47] Department of Veterans Affairs, Office of Inspector General, Health Care Inspection: Community Based Outpatient Clinic Reviews, Report No. 09-01446-233, Washington, DC, September 30, 2009. Department of

Veterans Affairs, Office of Inspector General, Health Care Inspection: Community Based Outpatient Clinic Reviews, Report No. 09-01446-226, Washington, DC, September 23, 2009. Department of Veterans Affairs, Office of Inspector General, Health Care Inspection: Community-Based Outpatient Clinic Reviews: Macon and Albany, GA, Beaver Dam, WI, Rockford, IL, Sioux City, IA, Aberdeen, SD, Waterloo, IA and Galesburg, IL, 09-01446-37, Washington, DC, December 2, 2009.

[48] Ashley N. Hedeen et al., "VA Community-Based Outpatient Clinics, Quality of Care Performance Measures," Medical Care, vol. 40, no. 7 (July 2002), pp. 570-577.

[49] Ibid. The Prevention Index is comprised of 9 performance indicators: immunization against influenza and pneumococcal diseases; tobacco use screening and cessation counseling; alcohol use screening; breast, cervical and colon cancer screening; and counseling regarding the risks and benefits of screening for prostate cancer. The Chronic Disease Care Index is comprised of 14 performance indicators for 5 common diagnoses: hypertension, diabetes mellitus, obesity, ischemic heart disease, and chronic obstructive pulmonary disease.

[50] Ashley N. Hedeen et al., "VA Community-Based Outpatient Clinics, Quality of Care Performance Measures," Medical Care, vol. 40, no. 7 (July 2002), p. 574.

[51] Ibid, p. 571.

[52] Chuan-Fen Liu et al., "The Impact of Contract Primary Care on Health Care Expenditures and Quality of Care," Medical Care Research and Review, vol. 65, no. 3 (June 2008), p. 311.

[53] John C. Fortney, Steven J. Borowsky, and Ashley N. Hedeen, et al., "VA Community-Based Outpatient Clinics: Access and Utilization Performance Measures," Medical Care , vol. 40, no. 7 (July 2002), pp. 561-569.

[54] Matthew L. Maciejewski, Michael K. Chapko, and Ashley N. Hedeen, et al., "VA Community-Based Outpatient Clinics: Cost Performance Measures," Medical Care, vol. 40, no. 7 (June 2002), pp. 587-595. Lower specialty and ancillary care costs may be lower due to CBOC providers becoming a "veteran's locus of care to avoid specialty and ancillary referrals," particularly when ancillary tests tend to be a cost driver.

[55] Department of Veterans Affairs, Veterans Health Administration, CBOC Performance Evaluation, Performance 2: Cost and Access Measures, Washington, DC, March 2002.

[56] Department of Veterans Affairs, Veterans Health Administration, CBOC Performance Evaluation, Performance 2: Cost and Access Measures, Washington, DC, March 2002.

[57] At present there are 21 VISNs (on January 23, 2002, the VA announced the merger of VISNs 13 and 14 into new VISN 23). Although VISNs are organized geographically, some VISNs cover more than one state, and some states are covered by more than one VISN.

[58] Department of Veterans Affairs, Office of Inspector General, Informational Report, Community-Based Outpatient Clinic Cyclical Reports, Report No. 08-00623-169, Washington, DC, July 16, 2009, p. 2.

[59] In October 2000, VA established the CARES program with the goal of evaluating the projected health care needs of veterans over the next 20 years and of realigning VA's infrastructure to better meet those needs. In August 2003, VA's Undersecretary for Health issued a preliminary Draft National CARES Plan (DNCP). Among other things, the draft plan called for the establishment of 48 new high-priority CBOCs.

[60] U.S. Congress, House Committee on Appropriations, Subcommittee on Military Construction, Veterans Affairs, and Related Agencies, Military Construction, Veterans Affairs and Related Agencies Appropriations for 2010, 111th Cong., 1st sess., 2009 (Washington: GPO, 2009), p. 1214.

In: Veteran Injuries, Disorders and Medical Care Service
Editors: Jessica Michaels and Jesse E. Levine
ISBN: 978-1-62081-302-7

Chapter 9

VETERANS' MEDICAL CARE: FY2012 APPROPRIATIONS*

Sidath Viranga Panangala

SUMMARY

The Department of Veterans Affairs (VA) provides benefits to veterans who meet certain eligibility criteria. Benefits to veterans range from disability compensation and pensions to hospital and medical care. The VA provides these benefits through three major operating units: the Veterans Health Administration (VHA), the Veterans Benefits Administration (VBA), and the National Cemetery Administration (NCA).

This report focuses on the VHA. The VHA is primarily a direct service provider of primary care, specialized care, and related medical and social support services to veterans through the nation's largest integrated health care system. Veterans generally must enroll in the VA health care system to receive medical care. Eligibility for enrollment is based primarily on previous military service, disability, and income. VA provides free inpatient and outpatient medical care to veterans for service-connected conditions and to low-income veterans for nonservice-connected conditions. The President submitted his FY2012 budget request to Congress on February 14, 2011.

The Administration's FY2012 budget request for VHA (medical services, medical support and compliance, medical facilities, and medical and prosthetic research) was $51.4 billion. The President's budget proposed to set up a $953 million contingency fund that would have provided additional funds up to $953 million to become available for obligation if the Administration determined that additional funds were required due to changes in economic conditions in 2012.

Furthermore, as required by the Veterans Health Care Budget Reform and Transparency Act of 2009 (P.L. 111-81), the President's budget requested $52.5 billion in advance appropriations for the three medical care accounts (medical services, medical support and compliance, and medical facilities) for FY2013.

On June 14, the House passed the Military Construction and Veterans Affairs and Related Agencies Appropriations bill (MILCON-VA Appropriations bill) for FY2012 (H.R.

* This is an edited, reformatted and augmented version of a Congressional Research Service publication, CRS Report for Congress R41944, from www.crs.gov, prepared for Members and Committees of Congress, dated January 6, 2012.

2055; H.Rept. 112-94). The House-passed measure provided $51.1 billion for VHA for FY2012. The Senate passed its version of the MILCON-VA Appropriations bill for FY2012 (H.R. 2055; S.Rept. 112- 29) on July 20. The Senate-passed version of H.R. 2055 provided a total of $51.2 billion for VHA. The House and Senate-passed versions of the MILCON-VA Appropriations bill for FY2012 provided $52.5 billion in advance appropriations for FY2013. Furthermore, both the House and Senate versions of the MILCON-VA Appropriations bill for FY2012 (H.Rept. 112-94; S.Rept. 112-29) did not approve the President's proposal to set up a $953 million contingency fund.

Congress did not pass the MILCON-VA Appropriations bill for FY2012 before the fiscal year began on October 1, 2011, and funded most of the VA through a series of short-term continuing resolutions (CRs).

On December 15, 2011, House and Senate conferees of H.R. 2055 reported a conference agreement (H.Rept. 112-331), which was titled the Consolidated Appropriations Act, 2012, and included nine appropriations bills. Division H of this measure contained the MILCONVA Appropriations Act, 2012. The Consolidated Appropriations Act, 2012 (P.L. 112-74; H.Rept. 112-331) was enacted into law on December 23, 2011. P.L. 112-74 provides a total of $51.2 billion for VHA for FY2012 and $52.5 billion in advance appropriations for FY2013. Consolidated Appropriations Act, 2012 (P.L. 112-74), did not approve the President's proposal to set up a $953 million contingency fund.

INTRODUCTION

The Department of Veterans Affairs (VA) provides a range of benefits and services to veterans[1] who meet certain eligibility rules; these benefits include medical care, disability compensation and pensions,[2] education,[3] vocational rehabilitation and employment services,[4] assistance to homeless veterans,[5] home loan guarantees, administration of life insurance as well as traumatic injury protection insurance for servicemembers,[6] and death benefits that cover burial expenses.[7]

The department carries out its programs nationwide through three administrations and the Board of Veterans Appeals (BVA). The Veterans Benefits Administration (VBA) is responsible for, among other things, providing compensation, pensions, and education assistance. The National Cemetery Administration (NCA)[8] is responsible for maintaining national veterans' cemeteries; providing grants to states for establishing, expanding, or improving state veterans' cemeteries; and providing headstones and markers for the graves of eligible persons, among other things. The Veterans Health Administration (VHA) is responsible for health care services and medical and prosthetic research programs. The VHA is primarily a direct service provider of primary care, specialized care, and related medical and social support services to veterans through the nation's largest integrated health care system. Veterans generally must enroll in the VA health care system to receive medical care. Eligibility for enrollment is based primarily on previous military service, disability, and income. Once enrolled, veterans are assigned to one of eight categories (see the *Appendix*). The VA provides free inpatient and outpatient medical care to veterans for service-connected conditions and to low-income veterans for nonservice-connected conditions.[9]

This report focuses on appropriations for VHA. It begins with a brief overview of the VA's budget for FY2011 (the current fiscal year) as a whole. It then presents a brief overview of VHA's budget formulation, description of the accounts that fund the VHA, and a summary of the FY2011 VHA budget. The report ends with a section discussing recent legislative developments pertaining to the FY2012 VHA budget.

Advance Appropriations[10]

In order to understand annual appropriations for the Veterans Health Administration (VHA), it is essential to briefly discuss the role of advance appropriations. In 2009, Congress enacted the Veterans Health Care Budget Reform and Transparency Act of 2009 (P.L. 111-81) authorizing advance appropriations for three of the four accounts that make up VHA: medical services, medical support and compliance, and medical facilities.[11] The fourth account, the medical and prosthetic research account, is not funded as an advance appropriation. P.L. 111-81 also required the Department of Veterans Affairs to submit a request for advance appropriations for VHA with its budget request each year. Congress first provided advance appropriations for the three VHA accounts in the FY2010 appropriations cycle. The Consolidated Appropriations Act, 2010 (P.L. 111-117), provided advance appropriations for FY2011, and the Department of Defense and Full-Year Continuing Appropriations Act, 2011 (P.L. 112-10), provided advance appropriations for FY2012.

Under current budget scoring guidelines, new budget authority for an advance appropriation is scored in the fiscal year in which the funds become available for obligation. Therefore, throughout the funding tables of this report, advance appropriations numbers are shown under the label "memorandum" and in the corresponding fiscal year column. For example, advance appropriations for FY2012 authorized by the Department of Defense and Full-Year Continuing Appropriations Act, FY2011 (P.L. 112-10), are shown under a separate memorandum and in the FY2012 column. However, it should be noted that budget authority for FY2012 refers to the budget authority authorized in P.L. 112-10 and any additional funding provided by the Consolidated Appropriations Act, 2012 (P.L. 112-74; H.Rept. 112-331) that includes funding for the medical and prosthetic research account (the account that is not funded as an advance appropriation).

Department of Veterans Affairs Budget

The VA's budget includes both mandatory and discretionary spending accounts. Mandatory funding supports disability compensation, pension benefits, education, vocational rehabilitation, and life insurance, among other benefits and services. Discretionary funding supports a broad array of benefits and services, including medical care. *Figure 1* provides a breakdown of FY2011 budget allocations for both mandatory and discretionary programs. In FY2011, the total VA budget authority was approximately $120.6 billion; discretionary budget authority accounted for about 47% ($56.3 billion) of the total, with about 86.3% of this discretionary funding going toward supporting VA health care programs, including medical and prosthetic research. The VA's mandatory budget authority accounted for about 53% of the total VA budget authority, with about 81% of this mandatory funding going toward disability compensation and pension programs.

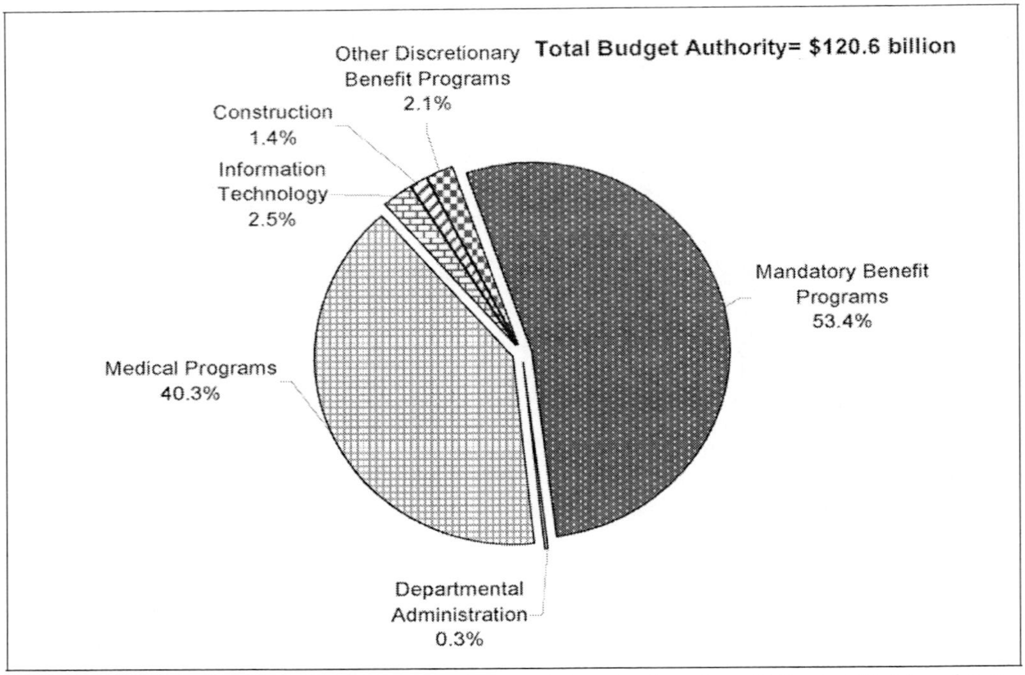

Source: Chart prepared by the Congressional Research Service based on H.Rept. 112-94 and S.Rept. 112-29.

Notes: Discretionary budget authority includes medical programs; information technology; construction; other discretionary benefits, such as operation and maintenance of VA's national cemeteries; and departmental administration.

Figure 1. FY2011 VA Budget Allocations.

Overview of Veterans Health Administration's Budget Formulation[12]

Similar to most federal agencies, the VA begins formulating its budget request approximately 10 months before the President submits the budget to Congress in early February. VHA's budget request to Congress begins with the formulations of the budget based on the Enrollee Health Care Projection Model (EHCPM).[13] The model estimates the amount of budgetary resources VHA will need to meet the expected demand for most of the health care services it provides.

The EHCPM's estimates are based on three basic components: the projected number of veterans who will be enrolled in VA health care, the projected utilization of VA's health care services—that is, the quantity of health care services enrollees are expected to use—and the projected unit cost of providing these services. Each component is subject to a number of adjustments to account for the characteristics of VA health care and the veterans who access VA's health care services. The EHCPM makes projections three or four years into the future based on data from the most recent fiscal year. For instance, in 2010, VHA used data from FY2009 to develop its health care budget estimate for the FY2012 request, including the advance appropriations request for FY2013.[14]

Funding for the VHA

As noted previously, VHA is funded through four appropriations accounts. These are supplemented by other sources of revenue. Although the appropriations account structure has been subject to change from year to year, the appropriation accounts used to support the VHA traditionally include medical care, medical and prosthetic research, and medical administration.

Congress also appropriates funds for construction of medical facilities through a larger appropriations account for construction for all VA facilities. In FY2004, "to provide better oversight and [to] receive a more accurate accounting of funds," Congress changed the VHA's appropriations structure.[15]

Specifically, the Department of Veterans Affairs and Housing and Urban Development and Independent Agencies Appropriations Act, 2004 (P.L. 108-199, H.Rept. 108-401), funded VHA through four accounts: (1) medical services, (2) medical administration (currently known as medical support and compliance), (3) medical facilities, and (4) medical and prosthetic research. Brief descriptions of these accounts are provided below.

Medical Services

The medical services account covers expenses for furnishing inpatient and outpatient care and treatment of veterans and certain dependents, including care and treatment in non-VA facilities; outpatient care on a fee basis; medical supplies and equipment; salaries and expenses of employees hired under Title 38, United States Code; cost of hospital food service operations;[16] and aid to state veterans' homes.

Medical Support and Compliance (Previously Medical Administration)

The medical support and compliance account provides funds for the expenses related to the administration of hospitals, nursing homes, and domiciliaries; billing and coding activities; public health and environmental hazard programs; quality and performance management; medical inspection; human research oversight; training programs and continuing education; security; volunteer operations; and human resources management.

Medical Facilities

The medical facilities account covers, among other things, expenses for the maintenance and operation of VHA facilities; administrative expenses related to planning, design, project management, real property acquisition and deposition, construction, and renovation of any VHA facility; leases of facilities; and laundry services.

Medical and Prosthetic Research

As required by law, the medical and prosthetic research program (medical research) focuses on research into the special health care needs of veterans.[17] This account provides funding for many types of research, such as investigator-initiated research; mentored research; large-scale, multi-site clinical trials; and centers of excellence. VA researchers receive funding not only through this account but also from the Department of Defense (DOD), the National Institutes of Health (NIH), and private sources.

In general, VA's research program is intramural; that is, research is performed by VA investigators at VA facilities and approved off-site locations. Unlike other federal agencies, such as NIH and DOD, VA does not have the statutory authority to make research grants to colleges and universities, cities and states, or any other non-VA entities.

Medical Care Collections Fund (MCCF)

In addition to direct appropriations accounts mentioned above, the Committees on Appropriations include medical care cost recovery collections when considering funding for the VHA. Congress has provided VHA the authority to bill some veterans and most health care insurers for nonservice-connected care provided to veterans enrolled in the VA health care system, to help defray the cost of delivering medical services to veterans.[18] Funds collected from First and Third Party (copayments and insurance) bills are retained by the VA health care facility that provided the care for the veteran.

As shown in *Table 1,* MCCF collections increased from $1.7 billion in FY2004 to $2.8 billion in FY2010. During this same period, first-party collections (for pharmacy, inpatient and outpatient, and long-term care copayments) increased by 17%, from $742 million to $870 million. In FY2004, first-party collections represented 42% of MCCF collections, and in FY2010, first-party collections represented approximately 31% of total collections. Furthermore, from FY2004 to FY2010, third-party collections increased by 98%, from $960 million in FY2004 to $1.9 billion in FY2010. In FY2004, third-party collections accounted for 55% of total collections, and in FY2010, third-party collections accounted for 67% of total MCCF collections.

FY2011 Budget Summary

President's Request

The Obama Administration released its FY2011 budget on February 1, 2010. The Administration's FY2011 budget request for three of the four accounts of VHA (medical services, medical support and compliance, medical facilities) was the same as the funding amounts provided in the MILCON-VA Appropriations Act of 2010 (P.L. 111-117), which was $48.1 billion. In addition, the President's request included $590 million for the medical and prosthetic research account. In total, the FY2011 budget request for VHA was $48.8 billion, excluding medical care collections. For FY2011, the Administration estimated that it will obtain $3.4 billion in medical collections, for a total VHA funding level of $52.1 billion. This is $4.1 billion, or 8.6%, above FY2010 levels (*Table 2*).

Furthermore, the President's budget requested $50.6 billion in advance appropriations for the three medical care accounts for FY2012. Specifically, the Administration's FY2011 budget request would have provided advance appropriations for FY2012 in the amount of $39.6 billion for the medical services account, $5.5 billion for medical support and compliance account, and $5.4 billion for the medical facilities account (*Table 2*).

House Action

On July 28, 2010, the House passed its version of the FY2011 Military Construction and Veterans Affairs and Related Agencies Appropriations bill (MILCON-VA Appropriations bill for FY2011, H.R. 5822; H.Rept. 111-559). The House-passed bill provided a total of $48.8 billion for the Veterans Health Administration (VHA) for FY2011, which included $48.1 billion authorized in the FY2010 Military Construction and Veterans Affairs and Related Agencies Appropriations Act (P.L. 111-117) and $590 million for the medical and prosthetic research account. H.R. 5822 provided advance appropriations of $50.6 billion for the medical services, medical support and compliance, and medical facilities accounts to be available in FY2012. This is the same as the Administration's request and 5.0% above the FY2011 total amount for the same three accounts (*Table 2*).

Senate Committee Action

On July 15, 2010, the Senate Committee on Appropriations marked up its version of the MILCON-VA Appropriations bill for FY2011 (S. 3615; S.Rept. 111-226). The Senate Appropriations Committee version of the bill provided $48.9 billion for VHA for FY2011. This amount includes $48.1 billion authorized in FY2010, an additional $120 million for the medical services and medical facilities accounts, and $590 million for the medical and prosthetic research account. The Senate Appropriations Committee-recommended amount was thus $120 million more than the President's request for VHA for FY2011. S. 3615 also provided an advance appropriation in the amount of $50.6 billion for medical services, medical support and compliance, and medical facilities accounts to be available in FY2012 (*Table 2*).

Full-Year Continuing Appropriations Act, 2011

At the beginning of the fiscal year, on October 1, 2010, FY2011 funding levels for most VA accounts had not been enacted by Congress. The three VHA accounts with advance appropriations were an exception.

Although the budget debate continued six months into the new fiscal year, funding for the medical services, medical support and compliance, and medical facilities accounts of VA had already been appropriated by the Consolidated Appropriations Act (P.L. 111-117, H.Rept.

111-366), which provided advance appropriations for these accounts. Therefore, these accounts were not affected by the series of continuing resolutions (CRs) passed by Congress.

On April 15, 2011, the President signed into law the Department of Defense and Full-Year Continuing Appropriations Act, 2011 (H.R. 1473, P.L. 112-10). This act provided a total of $52.0 billion for VHA for FY2011. This includes $48.6 billion in new budget authority and $3.4 billion in medical care collections (MCCF).

Additionally, P.L. 112-10 provided $50.6 billion in advance appropriations for FY2012 (*Table 2*).

Table 1. Medical Care Collections, FY2004-FY2010 ($ in thousands)

	FY2004 Actual	FY2005 Actual	FY2006 Actual	FY2007 Actual	FY2008 Actual	FY2009 Actual	FY2010 Actual
First-party pharmacy copayments[a]	$623,215	$648,204	$723,027	$760,616	$749,685	$720,238	$698,325
First-party copayments for inpatient and outpatient care	113,878	118,626	135,575	150,964	168,274	168,092	168,519
First-party long-term care copayments[b]	5,077	5,411	4,347	3,699	3,751	3,419	3,092
Subtotal first-party copayments	742,170	772,241	862,949	915,279	921,710	891,749	869,936
Third-party insurance collections	960,176	1,055,597	1,095,810	1,261,346	1,497,449	1,843,202	1,904,032
Enhanced use leasing revenue[c]	459	26,861	3,379	1,692	1,422	1,601	1,694
Compensated work therapy collections[d]	40,488	36,516	40,081	43,296	52,372	56,106	57,108
Parking fees[e]	3,349	3,443	3,083	3,136	3,355	3,585	3,611
Compensation and pension living expenses[f]	634	2,431	2,075	1,904	1,572	1,952	1,523
MCCF Total	$1,747,276	$1,897,089	$2,007,377	$2,226,653	$2,477,880	$2,798,195	2,837,904

Source: Department of Veterans Affairs, FY2012 Budget Submission, Medical Programs and Information Technology Programs, Volume 2 of 4, February 2011, pp. 1B-15.

Notes: The following accounts were not consolidated into the MCCF until FY2004: enhanced use leasing revenue, compensated work therapy collections, parking fees, and compensation and pension living expenses. Collection figures for these accounts for FY2003 are provided for comparison purposes.

[a]. In FY2002, Congress created the Health Services Improvement Fund (HSIF) to collect increases in pharmacy copayments (from $2 to $7 for a 30-day supply of outpatient medication; currently $8 for Priority Groups 2-6 veterans and $9 for Priority Groups 7 and 8 veterans), which went into effect on February 4, 2002. The Consolidated Appropriations Resolution, 2003 (P.L. 108-7)

granted the VA the authority to consolidate the HSIF with the MCCF and granted permanent authority to recover copayments for outpatient medications.

[b]. Authority to collect long-term care copayments was established by the Millennium Health Care and Benefits Act (P.L. 106-117). Certain veteran patients receiving extended care services from VA providers or outside contractors are charged copayments.

[c]. Under the enhanced-use lease authority, the VA may lease land or buildings to the private sector for up to 75 years. In return the VA receives fair consideration in cash and/or in-kind. Funds received as monetary considerations may be used to provide care for veterans.

[d]. The compensated work therapy program is a comprehensive rehabilitation program that prepares veterans for competitive employment and independent living. As part of their work therapy, veterans produce items for sale or undertake subcontracts to provide certain products and/or services, such as providing temporary staffing to a private firm. Funds collected from the sale of these products and/or services are deposited into the MCCF.

[e]. The Parking program provides funds for construction and acquisition of parking garages at VA medical facilities. The VA collects fees for use of these parking facilities.

[f]. Under the compensation and pension living expenses program, veterans who do not have either a spouse or child would have their monthly pension reduced to $90 after the third month a veteran is admitted for nursing home care. The difference between the veteran's pension and the $90 is used for the operation of the VA medical facility.

FY2012 VHA BUDGET

President's Request

The President submitted his FY2012 budget request to Congress on February 14, 2011. The Administration requested a total of $128.3 billion for the VA as a whole. This includes $69.5 billion in mandatory spending and $58.8 billion in discretionary spending (*Table 3*). The Administration's FY2012 budget request for VHA (medical services, medical support and compliance, medical facilities and medical and prosthetic research) is $51.4 billion.

In total, the FY2012 budget request for VHA is $54.6 billion, including medical care collections (*Table 4*). The President's budget is also proposing to set up a $953 million contingency fund that would provide additional funds up to $953 million to become available for obligation if the Administration determines that additional funds are required due to changes in economic conditions in 2012.

Funding for this contingency fund would be derived by revising the FY2012 advance appropriations request—included in the FY2011 President's budget request—by lowering the advance appropriations by $713 million to reflect the 2011 and 2012 estimated civilian pay freeze[19] and by requesting an additional $240 million for the medical services account in FY2012 (*Table 4*). Furthermore, the President's budget is requesting $52.5 billion in advance appropriations for FY2013 for the three medical care accounts (medical services, medical support and compliance, and medical facilities).

The President's budget request would provide $41.4 billion for the medical services account, $5.7 billion for the medical support and compliance account, and $5.4 billion for the medical facilities account (*Table 4*).

Table 2. VHA Appropriations by Account, FY2010-FY2011, and Advance Appropriations, FY2012
($ in thousands)

	Enacted (P.L. 111-117)		Request		House (H.R. 5822; H.Rept. 111-559)		Senate Committee (S. 3615; S.Rept. 111-226)		Full-Year Continuing Appropriations Act, 2011 (H.R. 1473; P.L. 112-10)[a]	
Account	FY2010	FY2011	FY2011[b]	FY2012	FY2011	FY2012	FY2011	FY2012	FY2011	FY2012
Medical Services	$34,707,500	—	$37,136,000	—	$37,136,000	—	$37,136,000	—	$37,061,728	—
Additional Funding over FY2011 Advance Appropriation	—	—	—	—	—	—	100,000	—	—	—
Subtotal Medical Services	34,707,500	—	37,136,000	—	37,136,000	—	37,236,000	—	37,061,728	—
Medical Support and Compliance (Previously Medical Administration)	4,930,000	—	5,307,000	—	5,307,000	—	5,307,000	—	5,296,454	—
Pay Freeze Rescission (P.L. 112-10)	—	—	—	—	—	—	—	—	-34,000	—
Subtotal Medical Support and Compliance (Previously Medical Administration)	4,930,000	—	5,307,000	—	5,307,000	—	5,307,000	—	5,262,454	—
Medical Facilities	4,859,000	—	5,740,000	—	5,740,000	—	5,740,000	—	5,728,550	—
Additional Funding over FY2011 Advance Appropriation	—	—	—	—	—	—	20,000	—	—	—

	Enacted (P.L. 111-117)		Request		House (H.R. 5822; H.Rept. 111-559)		Senate Committee (S. 3615; S.Rept. 111-226)		Full-Year Continuing Appropriations Act, 2011 (H.R. 1473; P.L. 112-10)[a]	
Account	FY2010	FY2011	FY2011[b]	FY2012	FY2011	FY2012	FY2011	FY2012	FY2011	FY2012
Pay Freeze Rescission (P.L. 112-10)	—	—	—	—	—	—	—	—	-15,000	—
Subtotal Medical Facilities	4,859,000	—	5,740,000	—	5,740,000	—	5,760,000	—	5,713,550	—
Medical and Prosthetic Research	581,000	—	590,000	—	590,000	—	590,000	—	579,838	—
Subtotal Medical and Prosthetic Research	581,000	—	590,000	—	590,000	—	590,000	—	579,838	—
Total VHA Appropriations (without collections)	45,077,500	—	48,773,000	—	48,773,000	—	48,893,000	—	48,617,570	—
Medical Care Cost Collections (MCCF)	2,954,000	—	3,393,000	—	3,393,000	—	3,393,000	—	3,393,000	—
Total VHA Appropriations (with collections)	$48,031,500	—	$52,166,000	—	$52,166,000	—	$52,286,000	—	$52,010,570	—
Memorandum: Advance Appropriations[c]										
Medical Services	—	$37,136,000	—	$39,649,985	—	$39,649,985	—	$39,649,985	—	$39,649,985
Medical Support and Compliance (Previously Medical Administration)	—	5,307,000	—	5,535,000	—	5,535,000	—	5,535,000	—	5,535,000
Medical Facilities	—	5,740,000	—	5,426,000	—	5,426,000	—	5,426,000	—	5,426,000

Table 2. (Continued)

	Enacted (P.L. 111-117)		Request		House (H.R. 5822; H.Rept. 111-559)		Senate Committee (S. 3615; S.Rept. 111-226)		Full-Year Continuing Appropriations Act, 2011 (H.R. 1473; P.L. 112-10)[a]	
Account	FY2010	FY2011	FY2011[b]	FY2012	FY2011	FY2012	FY2011	FY2012	FY2011	FY2012
Total VHA Advance Appropriations (without collections)	—	$48,183,000	—	$50,610,985	—	$50,610,985	—	$50,610,985	—	$50,610,985

Source: Prepared by the Congressional Research Service, based on figures from the Congressional Record, vol.171 (November 18, 2009), pp. S11503-S11508, Division E of H.Rept. 111-366; H.Rept. 111-559, and S.Rept. 111-226. FY2011 enacted figures based on information from the House Committee on Appropriations, Subcommittee on Military Construction, Veterans Affairs, and Related Agencies.

[a]. FY2011 enacted funding amounts reflects the 0.2% government-wide rescission required by Division B, Section 1119(a) of the Department of Defense and Full-Year Continuing Appropriations Act, 2011 (H.R. 1473, P.L. 112-10).

[b]. The President's Budget request for FY2011 reflects the same amounts appropriated for 2011in the MILCON-VA Appropriations Act of 2010 (P.L. 111-117) as an advance appropriation.

[c]. The Veterans Health Care Budget Reform and Transparency Act 2009 (P.L. 111-81; codified at 38 U.S.C. §117) provided for advance appropriations (appropriations that become available one fiscal year after the fiscal year for which the appropriations act was enacted) for VA's medical services, medical support and compliance, and medical facilities appropriations accounts, and requires the VA to submit a request for advance appropriation with its budget submission year.

Table 3. VA Appropriations, FY2011-FY2012, and Advance Appropriations, FY2013
($ in thousands)

	Full-Year Continuing Appropriations Act, 2011 (H.R. 1473; P.L. 112-10)		Request		House (H.R. 2055; H.Rept. 112-94)		Senate (H.R. 2055; S.Rept. 112-29)		Consolidated Appropriations Act, 2012 (P.L. 112-74; H.Rept. 112-331	
	FY2011[a]	FY2012	FY2012	FY2013	FY2012	FY2013	FY2012	FY2013	FY2012	FY2013
Total Department of Veterans Affairs	$120,641,583	—	$128,272,589	—	$127,796,852	—	$128,090,847	—	$122,226,272	—

	Full-Year Continuing Appropriations Act, 2011 (H.R. 1473; P.L. 112-10)		Request		House (H.R. 2055; H.Rept. 112-94)		Senate (H.R. 2055; S.Rept. 112-29)		Consolidated Appropriations Act, 2012 (P.L. 112-74; H.Rept. 112-331	
	FY2011[a]	FY2012	FY2012	FY2013	FY2012	FY2013	FY2012	FY2013	FY2012	FY2013
(VA)										
Total Mandatory	64,305,912	—	69,497,269	—	69,497,269	—	69,497,269	—	63,764,919	—
Total Discretionary	56,335,671	—	58,775,320	—	58,299,583	—	58,593,578	—	58,461,353	—
Total Veterans Health Administration (VHA)[b]	$48,617,570	—	$51,359,759	—	$51,141,759	—	$51,191,985	—	$51,191,985	—
Memorandum:										
Advance appropriations VHA[c]	—	$50,610,985	—	$52,541,000	—	$52,541,000	—	$52,541,000	—	$52,541,000

Source: Prepared by the Congressional Research Service. FY2011 enacted figures based on information from the House Committee on Appropriations, Subcommittee on Military Construction, Veterans Affairs, and Related Agencies, and S.Rept. 112-29. The FY2012 request and House and Senate figures are based on H.Rept. 112-94, and S.Rept. 112-29. Final enacted numbers for FY2012 based on H.Rept. 112-331.

[a]. This amount also reflects the 0.2% government-wide rescission required by Division B, Section 1119(a) of the Department of Defense and Full-Year Continuing Appropriations Act, 2011 (P.L. 112-10), and the FY2011 pay freeze rescission.

[b]. Includes funding for medical services, medical support and compliance, medical facilities, and medical and prosthetic research accounts, and excludes collections deposited into the Medical Care Collections Fund (MCCF).

[c]. The Department of Defense and Full-Year Continuing Appropriations Act, 2011 (P.L. 112-10) provided budget authority for FY2012 for the following accounts: medical services, medical support and compliance, and medical facilities. Under current budget scoring guidelines new budget authority for an advance appropriation is scored in the fiscal year in which the funds become available for obligation. Therefore, in this table the budget authority is recorded in the FY2012 column. Likewise, Consolidated Appropriations Act, 2012 (P.L. 112-74; H.Rept. 112-331) provided advance appropriations budget authority for FY2013 for those same accounts. Under current budget scoring guidelines, new budget authority for an advance appropriation is scored in the fiscal year in which the funds become available for obligation. Therefore, in this table this budget authority is recorded in the FY2013 column.

Table 4. VHA Appropriations by Account, FY2011-FY2012, and Advance Appropriations, FY2013
($ in thousands)

	Full-Year Continuing Appropriations Act, 2011 (H.R. 1473; P.L. 112-10)		President's Budget Request		House (H.R. 2055; H.Rept. 112-94)		Senate (H.R. 2055; S.Rept. 112-29)		Consolidated Appropriations Act, 2012 (P.L. 112-74; H.Rept. 112-331)	
Account	FY2011[a]	FY2012	FY2012	FY2013	FY2012	FY2013	FY2012	FY2013	FY2012	FY2013
Medical Services	$37,061,728	—	$39,649,985	—	$39,649,985	—	$39,649,985	—	$39,649,985	—
Additional Funding over FY2012 Advance Appropriation	—	—	$240,000	—	—	—	—	—	—	—
Subtotal Medical Services	37,061,728	—	39,889,985	—	39,649,985	—	39,649,985	—	39,649,985	—
Medical Support and Compliance (Previously Medical Administration)	5,296,454	—	5,535,000	—	5,535,000	—	5,535,000	—	5,535,000	—
Pay Freeze Rescission (P.L. 112-10)	-34,000	—	—	—	—	—	—	—	—	—
Subtotal Medical Support and Compliance (Previously Medical Administration)	5,262,454	—	5,535,000	—	5,535,000	—	5,535,000	—	5,535,000	—
Medical Facilities	5,728,550	—	5,426,000	—	5,426,000	—	5,426,000	—	5,426,000	—
Pay Freeze Rescission (P.L. 112-10)	-15,000	—	—	—	—	—	—	—	—	—
Subtotal Medical Facilities	5,713,550	—	5,426,000	—	5,426,000	—	5,426,000	—	5,426,000	—
Medical and Prosthetic Research	579,838	—	508,774	—	530,774	—	581,000	—	581,000	—
Subtotal Medical and Prosthetic Research	579,838	—	508,774	—	530,774	—	581,000	—	581,000	—
Total VHA Appropriations (without collections)	48,617,570	—	51,359,759	—	51,141,759	—	51,191,985	—	51,191,985	—
Medical Care Cost Collections (MCCF)	3,393,000	—	$3,326,000	—	3,326,000	—	3,326,000	—	3,326,000	—
Total VHA Appropriations (with collections)	$52,010,570	—	$54,685,759	—	$54,467,759	—	$54,517,985	—	$54,517,985	—
Memorandum: Advance										

	Full-Year Continuing Appropriations Act, 2011 (H.R. 1473; P.L. 112-10)		President's Budget Request		House (H.R. 2055; H.Rept. 112-94)		Senate (H.R. 2055; S.Rept. 112-29)		Consolidated Appropriations Act, 2012 (P.L. 112-74; H.Rept. 112-331)	
Account	FY2011[a]	FY2012	FY2012	FY2013	FY2012	FY2013	FY2012	FY2013	FY2012	FY2013
Appropriations[b]										
Medical Services	—	$39,649,985	—	$41,354,000	—	$41,354,000	—	$41,354,000	—	$41,354,000
Medical Support and Compliance (Previously Medical Administration)	—	5,535,000	—	$5,746,000	—	5,746,000	—	5,746,000	—	5,746,000
Medical Facilities	—	5,426,000	—	$5,441,000	—	5,441,000	—	5,441,000	—	5,441,000
Total VHA Appropriations	—	$50,610,985	—	$52,541,000	—	$52,541,000	—	$52,541,000	—	$52,541,000

Source: Prepared by the Congressional Research Service. FY2011 enacted figures based on information from the House Committee on Appropriations, Subcommittee on Military Construction, Veterans Affairs, and Related Agencies, and S.Rept. 112-29. FY2012 request and House and Senate figures based on H.Rept. 112-94, and S.Rept. 112-29. Final enacted numbers for FY2012 based on H.Rept. 112-331.

[a]. This amount also reflects the 0.2% government-wide rescission required by Division B, Section 1119(a) of the Department of Defense and Full-Year Continuing Appropriations Act, 2011 (P.L. 112-10), and the FY2011pay freeze rescission.

[b]. The Veterans Health Care Budget Reform and Transparency Act 2009 (P.L. 111-81; codified at 38 U.S.C. §117) provided for advance appropriations (appropriations that become available one fiscal year after the fiscal year for which the appropriations act was enacted) for VA's medical services, medical support and compliance, and medical facilities appropriations accounts, and requires the VA to submit a request for advance appropriation with its budget submission year. The Department of Defense and Full-Year Continuing Appropriations Act, 2011 (P.L. 112-10) provided budget authority for FY2012 for the following accounts: medical services, medical support and compliance, and medical facilities. Under current budget scoring guidelines new budget authority for an advance appropriation is scored in the fiscal year in which the funds become available for obligation. Therefore, in this table the budget authority is recorded in the FY2012 column. Likewise, the Consolidated Appropriations Act, 2012 (P.L. 112-74 (H.Rept. 112-331) provided advance appropriations budget authority for FY2013 for those same accounts. Under current budget scoring guidelines, new budget authority for an advance appropriation is scored in the fiscal year in which the funds become available for obligation. Therefore, in this table this budget authority is recorded in the FY2013 column.

House Budget Resolution

The House Budget Committee reported a concurrent resolution on the FY2012 budget (H.Con.Res. 34; H.Rept. 112-58) on April 11, 2011. The House passed H.Con.Res. 34 on April 15. According to the committee report accompanying H.Con.Res. 34 for veterans programs:

> The resolution calls for $128.3 billion in budget authority and $127.1 billion in outlays in fiscal year 2012. Discretionary spending, mainly veterans' health care, is $59.0 billion in budget authority and $57.9 billion in outlays in fiscal year 2012. This resolution also provides for up to $52.5 billion in advance appropriations consistent with the Veterans Health Care Budget and Reform Transparency Act of 2009. Mandatory spending in 2012 is $69.4 billion in budget authority and $69.3 billion in outlays.[20]

House Action

The House Military Construction and Veterans Affairs Appropriations Subcommittee approved a draft FY2012 Military Construction and Veterans Affairs and Related Agencies Appropriations bill (MILCON-VA Appropriations bill) on May 13, 2011. On May 24, the full House Appropriations Committee voted to report the measure. On June 14, the House passed the MILCON-VA Appropriations bill for FY2012 (H.R. 2055; H.Rept. 112-94). The House-passed bill provides a total of approximately $127.8 billion for the VA. This amount is 5.9% above the FY2011-enacted amount and $476 million below the FY2012 President's request (*Table 3*). The House-passed measure provides $51.1 billion for VHA for FY2012 (see *Table 4*). This is an increase of 5.2% over the FY2011-enacted amount and $218 million less than the President's request. Additionally, H.R. 2055, as passed by the House, provides $52.5 billion in advance appropriations for FY2013 for three relevant accounts (medical services, medical support and compliance, and medical facilities), the same amount as the Administration's request.

The bill also provides $531 million for the medical and prosthetic research account, a 4.3% increase over the President's request of $509 million (*Table 4).* The House-passed measure did not provide the additional $240 million requested by the President.

According to the committee report accompanying H.R. 2055:

> The Committee does not provide this additional FY 2012 funding. As the economy begins to recover, it seems unlikely that economic conditions will generate unmet medical services needs, particularly since the account has weathered the worst of the recession without budget shortfalls. The Committee's recommendation does not include rescission of $664,000,000 of FY 2011 and FY 2012 funding that remains in the medical care accounts from the cancelled pay raises. Rather, the Committee permits the funding to remain in the account to cover any unanticipated medical service costs. The bill includes language indicating that the $664,000,000 will be available only in the fourth quarter of the fiscal year upon approval of the Appropriations Committees of a request from the VA to release the funding due to unanticipated needs related to economic conditions.[21]

During floor debate of the MILCON-VA Appropriations bill, FY2012, Representative John Culberson offered H.Amdt. 409, which was agreed upon by the House. This amendment set aside $20 million from the medical services account for FY2012 for suicide prevention outreach.

Senate Action

On June 28, the Senate Appropriations Committee, Subcommittee on Military Construction, Veterans Affairs and Related Agencies marked up the FY2012 Military Construction, Veterans Affairs (VA) and Related Agencies Appropriations bill (MILCON-VA Appropriations bill, FY2012) and the full committee reported the measure with an amendment in the form of a substitute on June 30 (H.R. 2055; S.Rept. 112-29). The Senate passed the bill on July 20. The Senate-passed version of the MILCON-VA appropriations bill for FY2012 provides a total of approximately $128.1 billion for the Department of Veterans Affairs (VA) as a whole. This amount is 6.2% above the FY2011-enacted amount of $120.6 billion, and $182 million below the President's budget request of $128.3 billion (*Table 3).* The Senate–passed version of H.R. 2055 provides a total of $51.2 billion for VHA. This is a 5.3% increase over the FY2011-enacted amount and $168 million less than the President's request (*Table 4*). Similar to the House-passed version, the Senate-passed version of the MILCON-VA Appropriations bill, FY2012, provides $52.5 billion in advance appropriations for FY2013 for the three relevant accounts, the same as the Administration's request. The measure also provides $581 million for the medical and prosthetic research account, a 14.1% increase over the President's request and 9.4% increase over the House-passed amount for this account (*Table 4*). As was the case with the House-passed measure, the Senate bill did not provide the additional funding of $240 million or the $953 million contingency fund requested by the President. According to the Senate Appropriations Committee report:

> In addition to funding for VHA's regular Medical services programs, the Administration's budget submission requested a separate $953,000,000 contingency fund within the Medical services account in the event that the current economic climate results in a spike in veterans turning to the VA for their medical care. The request was partially offset by a rescission of $713,000,000 which was the cumulative 2011 and 2012 pay freeze. The balance, $240,000,000, was requested above the advance appropriation provided to the Department for fiscal year 2012. Under the proposal, the contingency funds would become available for obligation only if the Administration determined that additional funds were required due to unanticipated demand for VA medical services, and only if the Office of Management and Budget [OMB] approved the request. The Committee remains committed to providing the Department with every resource it requires to meet the needs of veterans, but it does not believe that the creation of a contingency fund, which takes control of medical resources out of the hands of the Department and places it within the jurisdiction of OMB, is prudent policy. Further, the Department's fiscal year 2013 request assumes that the VA will carry $500,000,000 over from fiscal year 2012. The Committee believes that before requesting a contingency fund the VA should utilize funding that is available to the Department. Toward this end, the Committee recommendation does not rescind $664,000,000 which remains in the medical care accounts from the cancelled pay raises, and rather leaves the funding within the

Medical services account for use by the Department to address unanticipated demand, should it materialize.[22]

Consolidated Appropriations Act, 2012

Congress did not pass the MILCON-VA Appropriations bill for FY2012 before the fiscal year began on October 1, 2011, and funded most of the VA through a series of short-term continuing resolutions (CRs)—P.L. 112-33, P.L. 112-36, P.L. 112-55, P.L. 112-67, and P.L. 112-68.[23] However, three of the four accounts—medical services, medical support and compliance, and medical facilities—that make up VHA were not affected since these accounts were provided advance appropriations in the Full-Year Continuing Appropriations Act, 2011 (P.L. 112-10).

On December 15, 2011, House and Senate conferees of H.R. 2055 reported a conference agreement (H.Rept. 112-331), which was titled the Consolidated Appropriations Act, 2012, and included nine appropriations bills. Division H of this measure contained the MILCON-VA Appropriations Act, 2012. [24] The Consolidated Appropriations Act, 2012 (P.L. 112-74; H.Rept. 112-331), was enacted into law on December 23, 2011. The measure provides a total of $122.2 billion for the Department of Veterans Affairs. This is a 4.7 % decrease from the President's request of $128.1 billion (*Table 3*). This change reflects the new budget estimates provided in the Administration's mid-session review.

The Consolidated Appropriations Act, 2012 (P.L. 112-74; H.Rept. 112-331), provides a total of $51.2 billion for VHA for FY2012. This is a 5.3% increase over the FY2011-enacted amount of $48.6 billion and 0.3% less than the President's request of $51.4 billion. The enacted amount includes $581 million for the medical and prosthetic research account, a 14.2 % increase over the requested amount of $509 million, and 9.5 % over the House-passed amount of $531 million (*Table 4*).

P.L. 112-74 also provides $52.5 billion in advance appropriations for FY2013 for three relevant accounts (medical services, medical support and compliance, and medical facilities), the same amount as the Administration's request (*Table 4*). The Consolidated Appropriations Act, 2012 (P.L. 112-74), did not approve the President's proposal to set up a $953 million contingency fund.

Appendix. VA Priority Groups and Their Eligibility Criteria

Table A-1. VA Priority Groups and Their Eligibility Criteria

Priority Group 1
Veterans with service-connected disabilities rated 50% or more disabling
Veterans determined by VA to be unemployable due to service-connected conditions

Priority Group 2

Veterans with service-connected disabilities rated 30% or 40% disabling

Priority Group 3

Veterans who are former POWsa

Veterans awarded the Purple Heartb

Veterans in receipt of the Medal of Honorc

Veterans whose discharge was for a disability that was incurred or aggravated in the line of duty

Veterans with service-connected disabilities rated 10% or 20% disabling

Veterans awarded special eligibility classification under Title 38, U.S.C., Section 1151, "benefits for individuals disabled by treatment or vocational rehabilitation"

Priority Group 4

Veterans who are receiving aid and attendance or housebound benefits Veterans who have been determined by VA to be catastrophically disabled Priority Group 5

Nonservice-connected veterans and noncompensable service-connected veterans rated 0% disabled whose annual income and net worth are below the established VA means test thresholds

Veterans receiving VA pension benefits

Veterans eligible for Medicaid benefits

Priority Group 6

Compensable 0% service-connected veterans

Mexican Border War veterans

Veterans solely seeking care for disorders associated with

—exposure to herbicides while serving in Vietnam; or

—ionizing radiation during atmospheric testing or during the occupation of Hiroshima and Nagasaki; or

—for disorders associated with service in the Gulf War; or

—for any illness associated with service in combat in a war after the Gulf War or during a period of hostility after November 11, 1998 as follows:

- Veterans discharged from active duty on or after January 28, 2003, who were enrolled as of January 28, 2008, and veterans who apply for enrollment after January 28, 2008, for five years post discharge

-Veterans discharged from active duty before January 28, 2003, who apply for enrollment after January 28, 2008, until January 27, 2011

Priority Group 7

Veterans who agree to pay specified copayments with income and/or net worth *above* the VA means test threshold and income *below* the VA national geographic income thresholds

Priority Group 8

Veterans who agree to pay specified copayments with income and/or net worth *above* the VA means test threshold and the VA national geographic threshold

Subpriority a: Noncompensable 0% service-connected and enrolled as of January 16, 2003, and who have remained enrolled since that date and/or placed in this subpriority due to changed eligibility status

Subpriority b: Noncompensable 0% service-connected and enrolled on or after June 15, 2009, whose income exceeds the current VA means test threshold or VA national geographic income thresholds by 10% or less

Table A-1. (Continued)

Subpriority c: Nonservice-connected veterans enrolled as of January 16, 2003, and who have remained enrolled since that date and/or placed in this subpriority due to changed eligibility status Subpriority d: Nonservice-connected veterans enrolled on or after June 15, 2009, whose income exceeds the current VA means test threshold or VA national geographic income thresholds by 10% or less Subpriority e: Noncompensable 0% service-connected veterans not meeting the above criteria Subpriority g: Nonservice-connected veterans not meeting the above criteria

Source: Department of Veterans Affairs.

Notes: Service-connected disability means with respect to disability, that such disability was incurred or aggravated in the line of duty in the active military, naval or air service.

Veterans who are former Prisoners of War (POWs) are placed in Priority Group 3. This change occurred with the enactment of the Former Prisoner of War Benefits Act of 1981(P.L. 97-37) on August 14, 1981.

Veterans in receipt of a Purple Heart are in Priority Group 3. This change occurred with the enactment of the Veterans Millennium Health Care and Benefits Act (P.L. 106-117) on November 30, 1999.

Veterans in receipt of the Medal of Honor are in Priority Group 3. This change occurred with the enactment of the Caregiver and Veterans Omnibus Health Services Act of 2010 (P.L. 111-163) on May 5, 2010.

End Notes

[1] In general, payments of benefits made to, or on account of, a beneficiary under any law administered by the VA are exempt from federal taxation (38 U.S.C. § 5301).

[2] For a detailed description of disability compensation and pension programs, see CRS Report RL34626, Veterans' Benefits: Benefits Available for Disabled Veterans, by Christine Scott and Carol D. Davis; CRS Report RL33323, Veterans Affairs: Benefits for Service-Connected Disabilities, by Douglas Reid Weimer; and CRS Report RS22804, Veterans' Benefits: Pension Benefit Programs, by Christine Scott and Carol D. Davis.

[3] For a discussion of education benefits, see CRS Report R40723, Educational Assistance Programs Administered by the U.S. Department of Veterans Affairs, by Cassandria Dortch.

[4] For details on VA's vocational rehabilitation and employment, see CRS Report RL34627, Veterans' Benefits: The Vocational Rehabilitation and Employment Program, by Christine Scott and Carol D. Davis.

[5] For detailed information on homeless veterans programs, see CRS Report RL34024, Veterans and Homelessness, by Libby Perl.

[6] For details on insurance programs, see CRS Report R41435, Veterans' Benefits: Current Life Insurance Programs, by Christine Scott.

[7] For details on death benefits, see CRS Report R41386, Veterans' Benefits: Burial Benefits and National Cemeteries, by Christine Scott.

[8] Established by the National Cemeteries Act of 1973 (P.L. 93-43).

[9] The term "service-connected" means, with respect to disability or death, that such disability was incurred or aggravated, or that the death resulted from a disability incurred or aggravated, in the line of duty in the active military, naval, or air service (38 U.S.C. § 101).

[10] In general, an appropriations act makes budget authority available beginning on October 1 of the fiscal year for which the appropriations act is passed ("budget year"). However, some types of appropriations do not follow this pattern; among them are advance appropriations. An advance appropriation means appropriation of new budget authority that becomes available one or more fiscal years beyond the fiscal year for which the appropriations act was passed (that is, beyond the budget year).

[11] Codified at 38 U.S.C. § 117.

[12] A major part of this discussion was drawn from U.S. Government Accountability Office, Veterans' Health Care: VA Uses a Projection Model to Develop Most of Its Health Care Budget Estimate to Inform the President's Budget Request, GAO-11-205, January 2011, pp. 4-8.

[13] The Veterans' Health Care Eligibility Reform Act of 1996 (P.L. 104-262) required the VHA to manage the provision of hospital care and medical services through an enrollment system based on a system of priorities.

[14] VHA uses methodologies other than the EHCPM to develop estimates of the amount of resources needed for longterm care services, and various legislative and health care related initiatives that may change from year to year.

[15] U.S. Congress, Conference Committees, Consolidated Appropriations Act, 2004, conference report to accompany H.R. 2673, 108th Cong., 1st sess., H.Rept. 108-401, p. 1036.

[16] In its FY2008 budget request to Congress, the VA requested the transfer of food service operations costs from the medical facilities appropriations to the medical services appropriations. The House and Senate Appropriations Committees concurred with this request. The cost of food service operations support hospital food service workers, provisions, and supplies related to the direct care of patients.

[17] 38 U.S.C. § 7303(a)(3). The Office of Research and Development (ORD) within the Veterans Health Administration (VHA) manages the medical research program. The medical research program encompasses, among other things, biomedical laboratory research, clinical trials, health services research, and rehabilitation research.

[18] The Consolidated Omnibus Budget Reconciliation Act of 1985 (P.L. 99-272), enacted into law in 1986. This law also established means testing for veterans seeking care for nonservice-connected conditions. The Balanced Budget Act of 1997 (P.L. 105-33) gave the VHA the authority to retain these funds in the Medical Care Collections Fund (MCCF). Instead of returning the funds to the Treasury, the VA can use them, without fiscal year limitations, for medical services for veterans. In FY2004, the Administration's budget requested consolidating several existing medical collections accounts into one MCCF. The conferees of the Consolidated Appropriations Act of 2004 (H.Rept. 108-401) recommended that collections that would otherwise be deposited in the Health Services Improvement Fund (former name), Veterans Extended Care Revolving Fund (former name), Special Therapeutic and Rehabilitation Activities Fund (former name), Medical Facilities Revolving Fund (former name), and the Parking Revolving Fund (former name) should be deposited in MCCF. The Consolidated Appropriations Act of 2005 (P.L. 108-447, H.Rept. 108-792) provided the VA with permanent authority to deposit funds from these five accounts into the MCCF.

[19] On November 29, 2010, the President proposed a freeze in civilian pay for federal employees for 2011 and 2012. The White House, Office of the Press Secretary, "Fact Sheet: Cutting the Deficit by Freezing Federal Employee Pay," November 29, 2010, http://www. whitehouse.gov/the-press-office/2010/11/29/fact-sheet-cutting-deficit-freezingfederal-employee-pay.

[20] U.S. Congress, House Committee on the Budget, Concurrent Resolution on the Budget-FY2012, report to accompany H.Con.Res. 34, 112th Cong., 1st sess., April 11, 2011 (Washington: GPO, 2011), p. 115.

[21] U.S. Congress, House Committee on Appropriations, Military Construction, Veterans Affairs, and Related Agencies Appropriations Bill 2012, report to accompany H.R. 2055, 112th Cong., 1st sess., May 31, 2011, H.Rept. 112-94, p. 37.

[22] U.S. Congress, Senate Committee on Appropriations, Military Construction and Veterans Affairs, and Related Agencies Appropriations Bill, 2012, report to accompany H.R. 2055, 112th Cong., 1st sess., June 30, 2011, S.Rept. 112-29, p. 41.

[23] For further information on the continuing resolutions see, CRS Report RL30343, Continuing Resolutions: Latest Action and Brief Overview of Recent Practices, by Sandy Streeter.

[24] The eight other appropriations bills that were included in this omnibus measure are: Division A–Department of Defense Appropriations Act, 2012; Division B–Energy and Water Development Appropriations Act, 2012; Division C–Financial Services and General Government Appropriations Act, 2012; Division D–Department of Homeland Security Appropriations Act, 2012; Division E–Department of the Interior, Environment, and Related Agencies Appropriations Act, 2012; Division F–Departments of Labor, Health and Human Services, and Education, and Related Agencies Appropriations Act, 2012; Division G–Legislative Branch Appropriations Act, 2012; and Division I–Department of State, Foreign Operations, and Related Programs Appropriations Act, 2012.

INDEX

#

A

B

D

E

F

G

H

N

O

T

U

V

W

Y